AF544965

ADVENTURE IN A WHEELCHAIR

Pioneering for the Handicapped

by

IDA DALY

with

Hazel Flagler Begeman

WHITMORE PUBLISHING COMPANY

Philadelphia

ISBN 0-87426-031-0
Library of Congress Catalog Card Number: 73:76735
Printed in the United States of America

To all the perceptive individuals, both handicapped and able-bodied, who had faith in our dreams and helped to implement them.

TABLE OF CONTENTS

FOREWORD

My Able Disabled Sister

Many handicapped persons have left a listless world to lead an active life through the help of my sister, Ida Flagler Daly. As a founder and director of the Seattle Handicapped Center, she has crisscrossed America and Europe in her efforts to gain understanding and support for the physically disabled.

Her most influential role is that of example. She is severely disabled herself, yet her life is busy and stimulating. She is a vibrant, ageless person with an ingrained optimistic outlook. Working with a Board of nine handicapped members having, as she points out, "one good leg, six good hands and nine good heads," she inspires a recreational oasis for several hundred who might otherwise be bored, depressed or discouraged.

In addition to developing the Seattle Handicapped Center, one of only a few in this country to be both financed and operated by the physically disabled themselves, she has led a long struggle for specialized housing, and was instrumental in securing the construction of the first high-rise apartment designed solely as housing for the physically handicapped, enabling them to live independently.

Ida was stricken at the age of four with a puzzling illness later diagnosed as muscular dystrophy. Our father was an active homesteader in the pioneering sense, and restlessly moved mother and six children from Iowa to Idaho, from Spokane, Washington, to Seattle. The adjustments were often hard on all of us, but perhaps this adventuresome life challenged Ida. Through the years, as she has gradually lost muscle strength, I have watched her take up harder tasks to complete—a college education, a library or club to organize, an arduous trip—each would test her will to persist.

In her younger days, MD was an unknown attacker, and doctors could only recommend "rest and nourishing food," massage, manipulation, steam baths and cold showers—all with hope but little or no progress toward recovery. As a mothering older sister, I felt her crises were my concern.

Ida's love of learning and the realization that her life was different motivated her in early high school years to aim for the development of what she had—a good mind, art talent, energy and an overwhelming desire to be independent and self-supporting.

In her college years, she carried a full curriculum, overcoming useless hands and weakened muscles with the help of friends and relatives who at times carried her bodily to classes. When our family decided to move from Seattle to a fruit ranch on the Columbia River, Ida begged to be left behind, insisting that she could manage by herself. Manage she did. She turned an old house into apartments and found that there was always someone happy to help for a lower rent.

During the depression of the thirties, Ida pursued her studies, developed a circle of friends. She became a serious art student, although painting was increasingly difficult. She would hold the brush with both hands, pushing the strokes from her shoulders, A one-man show of fifty paintings brought encouragement and financial rewards.

Her life changed one day when Frank Daly came to visit a friend in the apartment. Frank returned often to help with needed repairs and to take her for rides. In 1944, they were married. They loved to travel and tucked Ida's wheelchair into the car to explore California, Texas and Mexico.

As more muscles weakened, Ida turned her attention from painting to a club for the handicapped. One obligation she assumed was writing for the club publication, which she now edits. With better communication, the membership grew in numbers until a building was established and the Seattle Handicapped Center evolved. Ida became the director-in-residence—"the lady on the spot," as she was called. She was the catalyst who ten years later would involve the mayor and city council of Seattle, the Housing Authority, the Foundation, volunteers and citizens to spearhead her fantastic drive to construct a 150-unit high-rise apartment free of architectural barriers and designed to accommodate wheelchairs or any other unusual need of a handicapped person—the first of its kind in this country.

It was at this point in Ida's life that I began to see clearly how all the pieces fitted together——her early trials, the development of her talents and her inquisitive mind, and the courage to keep herself from falling by the wayside, her tremendous urge to be independent of relatives and friends. By 1965, she had received the Certificate of Distinguished Service to the Community from the Seattle Chamber of Commerce, and had twice been awarded the National Award from the President's Committee on Employment of the Handicapped "Washington State's Handicapped American of the Year."

There were other awards, too. One in particular, "Woman of Achievement" at the Matrix Table banquet in 1968, put a few extra adjectives near her name: "Undaunted by life, ceaseless and imaginative in her attack on its problems, ever optimistic, she is an effective executive and a sparkling example of the Courageous Woman at her finest." Ida was also named "Quadriplegic of the Year" by the *Toomey J. Gazette, International*, and cited for service to the Muscular Dystrophy Association of America. She received the Governor's Award for the "Handicapped American of the Year." My little sister had already made quite a name for herself.

One of her friends, Paul Brown, once said that whenever he thought of Ida he was reminded of the lines in Edmund

Cooke's poem:

> You are beaten to earth? Well, well, what's that?
> Come up with a smiling face.
> It's nothing against you to fall down flat,
> But to lie there—that's disgrace.

Ida finally consented to let me put her story in writing only because she felt it might help others.

Hazel Flagler Begeman

Austin, Texas
February, 1973

ADVENTURE IN A WHEELCHAIR

Chapter 1

IOWA CHILDHOOD—PUZZLING ILLNESS

From my wheelchair in my comfortable barrier-free home in Center Park Apartments I watch the myriad twinkling lights on one of Seattle's thickly settled hills and contemplate, with inner amazement, my new situation. The building itself seems a dream castle, being a modern seven-story "high-rise," designed specifically for people in wheelchairs. A second astounding fact is that I, who have been a quadriplegic for forty years, am a Management Aide. No words can express my joy at being a part of this great pioneering adventure! Hardships, disappointments, extreme efforts were all worthwhile and now fade into insignificance.

Reviewing the steps which have led to this moment, and thinking of the many letters, from as far away as South Africa, asking "How did you do it?" makes me feel that perhaps sharing my adventures may bring inspiration to others whose lives also must be commanded by their own efforts. So here is my story!

One of six children in an eight bedroom home in Cedar Falls, Iowa, my earliest memories are of playing in our spacious yard and on the Iowa State Teachers College campus across the street. We had a small acreage nearby where, in season, we picked strawberries, cut great bunches of purple grapes and gathered watermelons. Dad took us for rides in the "Surrey with the Fringe on Top." Mother, holding our baby brother tightly in her arms, was handsome in her hat with bird and veil, which enhanced her brown eyes.

Then, when I was four, came the illness from which I

couldn't seem to recover. Things happened that puzzled me. Playing one day with my little doll in her bed, I fell, crushing both. Later in the winter while riding on a bobsled, my mittens remained frozen to the sled as I fell off. I had no grip in my hands. I remember that mother picked me up in her arms, saying, "Something is wrong." A search for help began, but it always failed and only many years later did I learn that I had muscular dystrophy.

Dad, always a pioneer at heart, decided to "prove-up" on a homestead in Idaho. Of the children, only my two brothers and I were to go. The three-day train ride was quite an adventure. Many people carried lunches, and the coaches had a mingled aroma of dust and orange peel. Staying in one room over a store in Wendell, Idaho, was quite different from our big house, but I liked the closeness to mother and dad, who bought us marshmallow horseshoes covered with chocolate at the little shop below.

After a few days, we drove across the flat prairie to our homestead which, to become ours, had to be lived on for three months. There was just one building, a new barn, the front of which was painted white. Only the granary was floored. This was to be our home for the hot summer of 1909.

With grub hoes and strong, gloved hands, dad and a hired man worked long hours every day, clearing the land. Huge bonfires of sagebrush lighted the area every night. One Sunday we had a trip in the wagon down into the Snake River Canyon—a steep, winding road. A man on horseback rode ahead "to kill the rattlesnakes," dad explained. Though the day was hot, I was wearing long underwear and black stockings because our Dr. Meade advised it! I fell while in the canyon, but not wanting to admit weakness, I waited until we returned home to tell mother. I still have a scar from the gash.

On May Day, my brothers and I carried our carefully made May baskets on a long walk across the prairie to a neighbor's house. We found bedlam raging among the children, but surprised silence came when they saw the baskets full of homemade fudge. May baskets were a Midwest custom, unknown "out West" at that time.

In retrospect, I imagine that mother's life was not easy there. Sand was a problem; each night it drifted in front of our door until it would scarcely open. Water had to be carried into the house from barrels hauled from a distant well. The altitude played havoc with her bread recipe, causing it to rise alarmingly until it touched the scorching sides of the oven.

As a reward for homesteading, dad took us to the Alaska Yukon Pacific Fair in Seattle. I remember only the Forestry Building, the turnstiles and streetcars.

We returned by train to our Midwest home only to pack up and leave for another pioneering venture—a new fruit farm in Emmett, Idaho, planted on virgin soil and watered by the new Canyon canal.

Left much to myself and being inactive, I felt an impulse to create something. In the packing shed I found some large shingles and some blue and white house paint. Because the colors suggested marine scenery, I painted lakes and oceans. I'm sure they were terrible, but they led to painting lessons with Mrs. Cook, a remarkable artist who lived nearby.

I was of school age now and my older sisters, who also painted under Mrs. Cook's direction, were most helpful. One result was my painting of the headwaters of the Canyon Canal (our irrigation project). It was hung in the Idaho Building of the San Francisco World's Fair. Several school chums and I started an art club. We papered the walls of an old shed and decorated them with magazine pictures of Greek ancient ruins. I was happy to be part of a gang, doing things I could do, for already the feeling of "being different" was developing.

Our fruit farm was outside of town about three miles, near the foothills. One morning when I was fourteen, I felt unusually strong and had an urge to test my strength. Behind our house there was a hill with three humps. I climbed the first as easily as anyone, much to my astonishment. I climbed the second hump and looked back, amazed at what I had done. I ran home fast, kicking up my heels, and I didn't feel the least bit tired. It was an unexplained thrust of strength; three days later, when I tried to climb the hill again, I couldn't make the first hump.

It was then I knew for sure that my life would be different. I walked every day, hoping to gain strength, but no progress was evident when I entered school in September. Studies were a joy—activities too much for me. Because of architectural barriers, it took 12 years for me to finish high school!

In this small town, all elementary classes were on the first floor. High school rooms were up one flight. There was a railing and, with considerable effort, I was able to get up the steps. Our home had no steps and no one in the family realized how weak I had become until one morning my sister Hazel, who was a teacher on the first floor, saw me laboring to climb. Later she told me she went back to her classroom, put her head down on the desk and cried. The next year, study hall was moved to the third floor and I was forced to give up until I was eighteen, when my father, ever mindful of my condition and the educational limitations of the small community, decided to move to a larger city. Because it was midway between Emmett and his Canadian wheatland, he chose Spokane, Washington. Here he bought a lovely home and returned to the fruit farm for the family. A new adventure had begun for me.

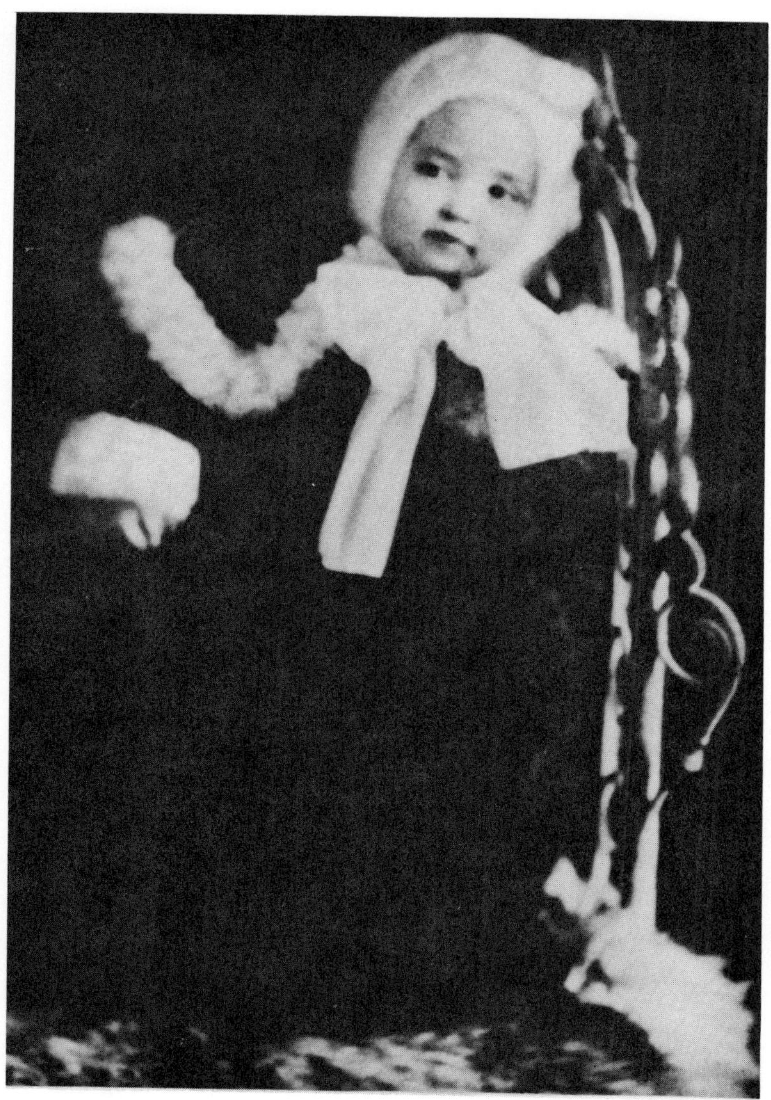

I was a healthy baby. Then, when I was four, came the illness from which I couldn't seem to recover.

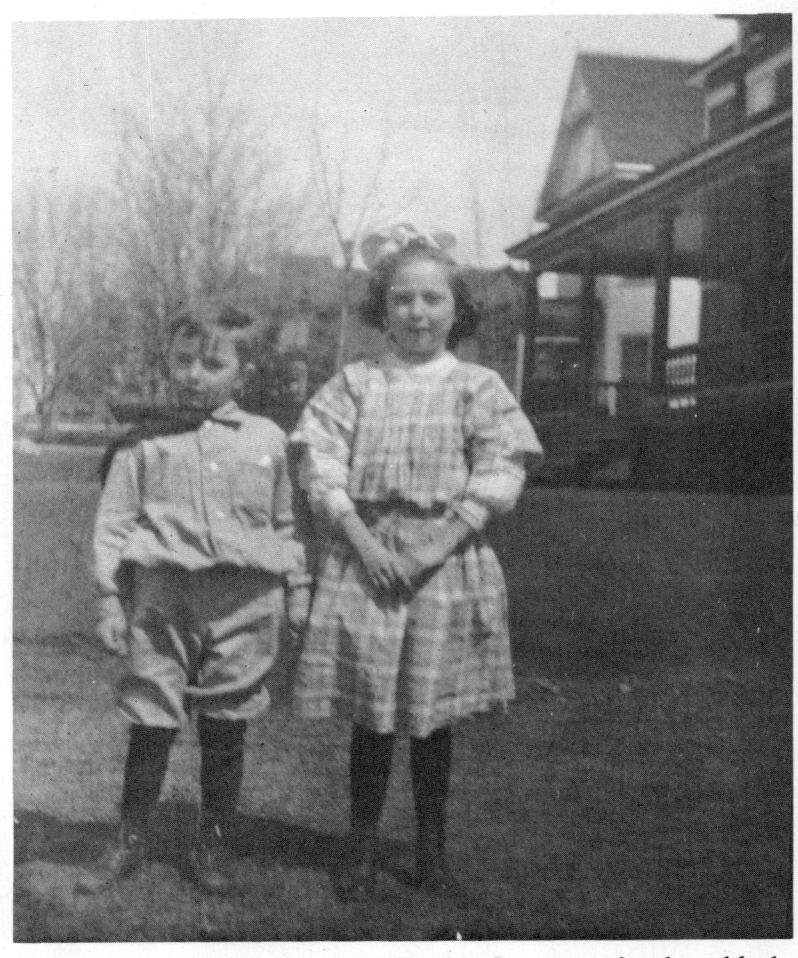

Here, playing with my brother, Charles, I was wearing long black stockings, which Dr. Meade advised, even though the day was hot!

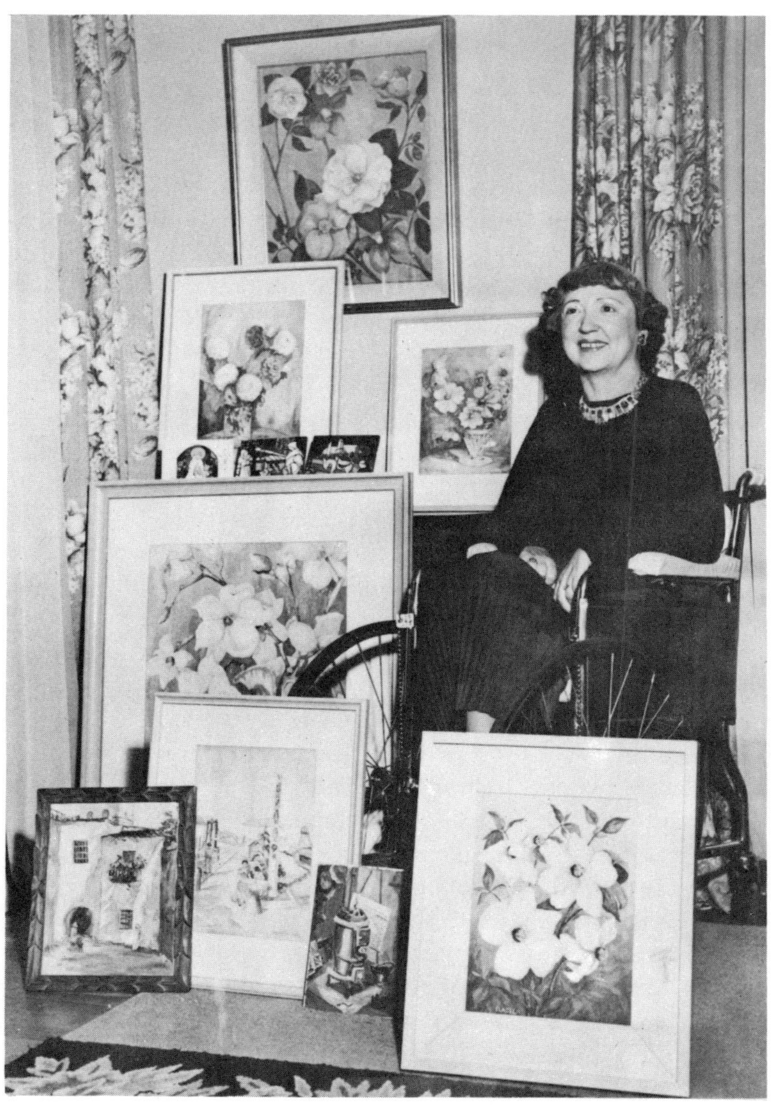

The painting, "Pink Dogwood," was one of several I made from one spray brought to me by a friend.

Chapter 2

TEENAGE OBSTACLES

Arriving by train, we were met by the Davenport Hotel bus, which I remember opened in the rear. The hotel lobby looked like an out-of-door patio with a red brick floor. In the middle was a wishing well, and around the room were ivy-covered latticed booths.

After lunch dad took us to our new home—three stories, like the one of my early childhood. The ceiling of the living room was beamed and there was a huge lava rock fireplace at one end. I loved my room with its beautiful brass bed, white dressing table and matching desk. This room still appears in my dreams occasionally.

Though my illness had no name as yet, a nerve specialist treated me with vibrator and electric pads which neither helped nor harmed. I was interested only in going to high school. Lewis and Clark High had several steps leading to the class level, but with the help of my brother, I was able to climb them. Since the cafeteria was on the next floor, I carried raisins and nuts for lunch which I ate in rather lonely isolation in any empty room, hoping no one would notice me. I here began the practice which determined my entire education, that of taking whatever classes were on the first floor. Soon after my return to high school, I felt my strength had drained away. Later, when I had recovered somewhat, my brother helped me and I finished that school year. But it was not until several years later, when an elevator was installed, that I could complete required courses and graduate with my "baby" sister, Marion, who was 10 years younger than I. As a reward for my persistence, mother gave me her most prized possession—a pearl-studded lapel watch.

One morning while dressing I fell. Mother heard the thud and came in to pick me up. I leaned against the warm radiator to steady myself, and concentrated on a picture in order not to cry. For a week I was in bed completely helpless. Muscles of my throat were affected and I could manage only liquids. The day before Easter I felt that if Christ were especially close to earth on that day, as depicted in the long poem I had memorized, "King Robert of Sicily," perhaps He would help me. Next day I was better and able to walk, but the use of my hands did not return.

Now there was a new doctor—more massages, manipulation, steam baths and cold showers. I still could not write or make the pen-and-ink sketches in which I had taken so much pride.

At this time, I found a new friend who herself had faced life as an invalid. She saved herself with what psychologists call "power of suggestion and the directing of the subconscious mind." She believed that the intelligent repetition of the same idea on the same mind would bring results. The concept had a tremendous impact on my whole being, though I did not expect the sudden physical change which occurred. Energy poured through me so fast that my hands trembled and my legs quivered. My doctor could not explain it. On the following Sunday, I walked to church—several blocks up a steep hill covered with snow. I helped a woman who had fallen, then walked up the steps of the church without touching the rail. On following days I could play runs and chords on the piano, clear the table of dishes and wipe silverware. Now terrifically happy, it seemed to me that I had been in a dark well and that now the top was taken off, revealing the sky.

Such spurts of strength were short-lived. My normal gait, prior to my need for a wheelchair, was slow and rather like a real-life rag doll. We still didn't know what was wrong, so I decided to seek more advanced medical expertise in St. Louis, where Hazel and her family were living.

Chapter 3

ADVENTURE IN ST. LOUIS

Hazel and her husband, ever ambitious for me, urged me to make my home with them for a while and attend classes at Washington University. I felt the change in environment would give me a new personality. I might lose my shyness and speak with greater ease. Then, too, there was hope of treatment by doctors in a large city. The barrier of steps decreed my college courses, too. At Washington University in St. Louis, I elected to major in Spanish because it was the most accessible class. Perhaps I could become self-supporting by tutoring Spanish was my thought at the time.

My sister's husband took me to the university for night classes, often carrying me upstairs. Though I could walk alone, it was difficult. I could negotiate stairs only by using both hands on the rail to pull myself up. We would all go to the art museum in Forest Park. I'll never forget the glass exhibit from Sweden, the Persian rugs, the French Impressionists, and the Chinese porcelains.

Other St. Louis memories are the New York Theatre Guild, opera in Forest Park, and the excursion boat trips on the Mississippi with my sister's family.

My sister made an appointment for me to enter Barnes Hospital. The head of the orthopedic section talked to me first. He called in a neurologist. Over a period of nine days, I had twelve doctors. Photographs and X-rays were made. Dr. Schwab gave me the news: progressive muscular dystrophy. No need for any treatments—just rest and nourishing food.

So I knew that my life was to be just what I could make of it from day to day. Long range planning was out. I would never marry, I told myself, so I must find a way to be independent. A short time later, I suffered a severe cold with high fever. For a few days afterwards, I could walk upstairs and around the yard. So very puzzling! This reaction to fever was to persist for many years. None of the doctors we questioned could explain.

Chapter 4

PAINTING BECOMES MY PASSION

After two years in St. Louis, I returned to Spokane, stopping on the way to see my childhood home in Iowa. I found the "steep terraces," down which my brother and I had daringly rolled, not so steep, the built-in kitchen table with the zinc top that had looked as big as a battleship to my child eyes, now just ordinary sized.

When I got home, I begged dad to move to Seattle so that I could continue university classes. It didn't take too much urging. My father loved the water, and he was ready to move again. He chose a home for us near Lake Union and a yacht club. Not knowing how I would manage, I enrolled in the University of Washington for art, sociology and Spanish classes. I could still walk, but only with much effort. My younger sister carried my books and drove me to the university; a friend's husband helped me up the steps at Denny Hall. The greatest happiness came to me here. I made real friends—a group of seven or eight who gathered around our fireplace for wonderful conversations. One of the "gang," Hector Chevagny later became blind and wrote a book, *My Eyes Have a Cold Nose*. He later did radio work in New York and was an inspiration to me. Another friend, Kenneth Calahan, became a prominent Northwest artist.

Another avenue of enjoyment was opened one night by a guest professor who noticed my watercolor paintings and asked why I was not specializing in that department. I looked at my useless hands for the answer. Understanding, he replied, "You do not paint with your hands, but with your eyes, mind and emotion. It doesn't matter how you hold your brush, by hands, teeth or toes."

Next day he brought me tubes of the three primary colors, and a small flat sable brush. He showed me how to put the paints on the pallette and mix them. Then he left me to discover *how*. Since I had been writing by grasping my pen in *both* hands, using a free arm movement from muscles in my shoulders and back, it seemed logical to use the brush in the same way. To my delight it worked! I first copied a scene from a postcard, next a Persian mosque from *National Geographic*. I painted on cardboard from the backs of tablets, on old window shades and scraps of wall board. These were depression days.

Since I had never seen anyone paint in oils, I studied from books at the library. Friends liked my flower paintings and bought them, so I had money for canvases and began to paint landscapes as well as flowers.

Strangely enough, my subjects often came to me in dreams. One night I dreamed that I was riding horseback along a ridge of hills. I turned west through an opening in the hills and came upon a great flat valley, all in oranges, reds and yellows. There were many dark pools and a range of hills in the distance. A visiting artist from Boston was amazed at what I had done in recreating my dream on canvas with such a tiny brush.

I wanted to paint what I saw rather than dreamed, and was fortunate to have access to an old rundown house in which I later lived. Wearing my brother's wool pants for warmth, I may have been the forerunner of the pants craze! With help I got on the low garage roof. There I painted the rear of the two-story house. The balcony, an enclosed porch and a precipitous winding stairway made an interesting pattern of flat surfaces, angles and shadows. The painting was done on a large piece of three-ply veneer board, with some areas left unpainted to give old wood effects. Browns, blue and grays were used with gesso to cover the grain of the wood. A large cherry tree spread over all, but I simplified the design by using only the trunk and a few bare branches.

So as to have some comparison with other painters, I decided to submit this painting to the Western Washington State Fair Exhibit. I was awarded first prize! That was the encouragement I needed, and with renewed ambition, I painted constantly and won several other awards.

The depression had ended my college days shortly before graduation. By the time funds were again available, I had been forced into a wheelchair by the progressing dystrophy, and, since my interest had turned to art and later to working for the Handicapped Club, I did not return to complete the last year of college. [In 1969, when I took on the post of Program Development for the Center Park Apartments for the Handicapped, I reentered college to take five hours of Sociology and bring myself up-to-date in the field. It was also a test of my ability to still study. Gratefully, I found academic work not only possible but most enjoyable. Perhaps someday, if I ever "retire," I may go after that degree.]

About this time, when the depression was at low ebb, mother and dad felt they must sell our Seattle home and live on the new fruit ranch they were developing on the Columbia River in Central Washington. On a dark, rain drenched day in January, 1933, we moved into a downstairs apartment of the "old rundown house." A few months later dad and mother went back to the ranch. I begged to be allowed to stay. The absentee owners needed someone to live there and send the rentals to them. I knew I could do that. I finally persuaded mother to leave me in the care of friends, who moved into the apartment with me when they left. The four-apartment old house near the university was a convenient location for married students. For the first time in my life I had a feeling of independence.

Chapter 5

INDEPENDENT AT LAST!

So now I was manager of a four-unit apartment. Everything about the place needed repairs. Every wind brought a shower of decaying shingles off the roof, and large sections of eaves came crashing down in the night. Rents were low and tenants pitched in to solve our common problems. With wallpaper at eight cents a roll and all labor donated, the place was finally made habitable. It was at this point that I consented to swallow my pride and take to a wheelchair. I wanted to get around faster, although at times I was still strong enough to walk.

There always seemed to be an ambitious couple attending the university, glad to care for me in lieu of rent. A friend, Phyllis, whose husband had been called into the navy, heard through a mutual friend that I needed help. She wired me, "Do you have room for me and one small dog?" I would have taken on a whole kennel to get her! She soon had everything running smoothly. On warm days we would go out together in the little electric car (which my father financed) to parks and the University of Washington campus, where we sketched and painted. If I went out alone, Rags, her wise little Boston terrier, would meet me on my return and bound in to get Phyllis.

Phyllis was a good model, generous in posing, never sensitive. One day I sketched her curled up on my studio couch writing a letter to her husband in the South Pacific. I stylized her face and hair and painted in flat areas, cutting out all details except the couch with green cover and her red sweater. Titled "Air Mail Letter" it was accepted by a jury at Little Studio Gallery in the Medical Arts Building in downtown Seattle.

My sister sent me a carved frame from Mexico. Especially for it, I painted Phyllis as a Mexican woman with a blue shawl—a suggestion of a black iron gate leading to a church, calling it "La Pensarosa," the sorrowful one. Phyllis had an interesting face, long and narrow with beautiful luminous eyes and straight black hair.

One usually can find subjects from any window. Outside my studio on our neighbor's lawn there was a clothesline supported by Y-shaped posts. One day as I looked out, the lines were full of glistening white sheets. Two women in black dresses were taking them down hurriedly, ahead of a threatening storm. I sketched quickly and later made several oils of this interesting contrast of black and white.

Many subjects I chose were close at hand. I could see some from my window—"Our Wood Pile," "Old Cherry Tree," "Potted Red Begonia," "Chair with Trowel." "Pink Dogwood" was one of several floral pictures I painted from one spray brought to me by a friend.

It was during this time that I painted a large canvas of my parents from an old wedding photograph found in the attic. A letter from my aunt who had been at their wedding furnished the color of mother's dress. Secretly I worked on this from February until July, when I presented it to my parents on their fiftieth wedding anniversary. They were moved, and dad was especially impressed with the detail of mother's dress.

At a time when my strength was ebbing, my sister Lorna from nearby Suquamish invited me to have a one-man show—a benefit for her Orthopedic Guild. With the help of Hazel, (visiting from St. Louis) who matted and framed, we had fifty paintings ready. Happily for me and the Guild, many sold.

One year I decided to paint an entry to confound the judges. There was a large, round mirror on my painting table, another beveled mirror tilted on the wall, and across the room a third mirror above the fireplace. The table mirror reflected my painting equipment—vase of brushes, palette, easel in the foreground. The wall mirror with its reflection of the room included the fireplace mirror, which in turn had its own reflections. For this I received second prize at the State Fair, besides the fun of doing it!

At about this time, it became possible for me to attend art class at the Edison Vocational School. I was fortunate to be accepted in Edwin Burnley's portraiture class. He was an excellent teacher, and his selection of live models gave a wide variety of contrasts. There was a Greek flute player who, in his day, had played for royalty. He was an outstanding character on the streets of Seattle, wearing his long black cape and large wide-brimmed hat. The children loved him.

Other models were a Welsh miner with a fur cap above his red face with cheerful, squinty eyes; a granddaughter of Chief Seattle; a white Russian woman refugee in a ball gown of happier days; and a turbaned student from India. Once again I felt the joys of working as part of a group!

On one of the class nights, I took some flower paintings for criticism. Paul Immel's daughter happened to be visiting the class. She said I should be studying with her father, and asked to take them home. He was interested and wanted me for a pupil in his watercolor flower painting class. It was in his class that I learned flower arrangement and the way of blending colors for the background.

One experience leads to another—a well-recognized artist asked to bring her class to my studio. They cleared my table, which was 30 inches wide and 7 feet long, got two pails of water, and used O'Hara's method, running washes to keep the paint loose, wet and drippy. We met out-of-doors when it was warm, attracting onlookers. This group experience made me more confident with others.

Over a period of years I continued managing the apartments, always, of course, with the help of couples. Though the house was old, I realized that its location near the university was valuable. So I wrote to the out-of-town owner, making a modest offer for the property. Much to my delight, it was accepted and I found myself not only independent, but the owner of my own home with four apartments to rent. I often reflect how the darkest of days (when we had to leave the much loved home near the lake and move into the old apartments) had in the end brought me what I most fervently desired, the chance to be self-supporting.

Chapter 6

UNEXPECTED HAPPENING—MARRIAGE

Remember my youthful conviction that I would never marry? One never can predict the future! One day as I was painting at the front window, a car stopped and a man got out to visit friends in one of my apartments. He looked so kind and jolly that I felt I wanted to know him. We were introduced and he soon began inviting me out to dinner. Frank Daly didn't mind my being in a wheelchair or my unusual way of eating by holding my fork in both hands (the way I used my paintbrush). We would take long rides in his little Plymouth roadster around the lake and to Everett to see his sister, as well as to Tacoma to see my youngest sister, Marion, and her family. We heard Roland Hayes at the Metropolitan downtown and attended many ballets and plays on the campus.

Frank was a pharmacist and worked out of town. On weekends he came to Seattle and often helped me with needed repairs on the apartments. He strengthened my confidence in meeting people and said often that I helped him. February 28, 1944, on a lovely spring evening, in front of my fireplace with only a few friends present, we were married. This wheelchair marriage brought happiness and mutual benefit for the next fourteen years.

One day in the early 1950's, Frank's sharp ears caught a news broadcast about muscular dystrophy. It was Drew Pearson's radio news and a change in sponsor or some restrictive ruling prompted him to remark, "I can't talk about Dobbs Hats tonight, so I will discuss something else—a rare disease that is fatal to youngsters but is not being given much attention." He went on to say that only $10,000 was being spent annually on research, and that a New York University doctor was the only man studying it.

At about the same time, the *Saturday Evening Post* ran a story about the dystrophic sisters in Texas—the famous Woods sisters, who became nationally known for organizing the National Muscular Dystrophy Research Foundation.

Frank saw a small item in the paper inviting anyone interested to attend a meeting to discuss forming a Muscular Dystrophy Society. It was held in a home in Ballard. We joined that night and worked actively together in developing the group which later joined the national organization when it was formed in New York. At last MD had captured public interest; research was to be launched and families would be drawn together for mutual support.

Frank added many new horizons to my life. Greater mobility was one. Just as I was a forerunner of the pants craze, Frank was probably the first to make a shoulder strap for a car. Twice I had been pitched forward out of the seat when a stop was unavoidable—once when a little girl on roller skates wheeled directly in front of us. The experiments were many. Finally he used canvas webbing purchased at a tent and awning shop. At Sears he found a harness snap. The strap went under both arms and was easy to snap on and off the sturdy lap robe bar on the back of the seat. An improvised footrest, attached to the underside of the dashboard, afforded comfort and aid in my constant battle against contractures.

Now Frank was ready to prove to me that I could take trips longer than our rides around Seattle. One of the trial runs was over Snoqualmie Pass, then on to Blewett Pass, and home by Stevens Pass, about two hundred and fifty miles. It was a beautiful spring day. The mountain streams were all rushing torrents. The early foliage was yellow against a background of green pines.

To avoid unnecessary lifting in and out of the car, I prepared ahead for long trips by dehydrating my body. I allowed myself no liquids the evening before and for breakfast had only two segments of orange and a few sips of coffee with egg on toast. At noon we ate in the car—apples, cheese, dates and cookies. Late in the afternoon, Frank would bring me a drink of water so the dehydrating would not endanger my health. Through the years I have arranged many trips for the handicapped and have often wished they would give up their morning coffee on those days to make things easier for our volunteer helpers! Unless some health factor is critical, I do not believe going without liquids for part of a day would be injurious to anyone.

Marriage enabled me to have my first pet. Very often a pet can bring a happy diversion to a handicapped person. Let me tell you about Nubia. Everyone, I guess, has to avert the eyes from stray cats. I had for many years, but when Frank came in one morning and said, "You should see the beautiful black cat on our doorstep," I could only say, "Bring her in." She entered majestically, walked around the apartment, looking over the place as if to see if it met her standards of a home. She was a handsome animal with heavy, black seal-like hair. It was her little pointed face that endeared her to Frank. She had sharp ears with tufts of hair rising to a point, and a long plush-like tail. All this and her loud voice were marks of part-Siamese lineage. We fed her and she stayed. She flattered me and fawned over me the first few days—even sleeping on my bed, but once sure of her position, she recognized Frank as her friend and provider, paying no attention to me unless Frank was away at work. She met him each night, knowing some way just when he would return. One time when he had left her at the veterinarian's for several days, she greeted him with both paws held out like a child. Even the vet had never seen a cat do that before!

Frank's advent into my life brought many happy changes. The adjoining apartment still housed the family of whichever tenant was doing our housework and attending to me when he was away. Frank took over personal responsibilities, which helped me in extending my activities and increasing my productivity, for example, in painting. Frank now owned a

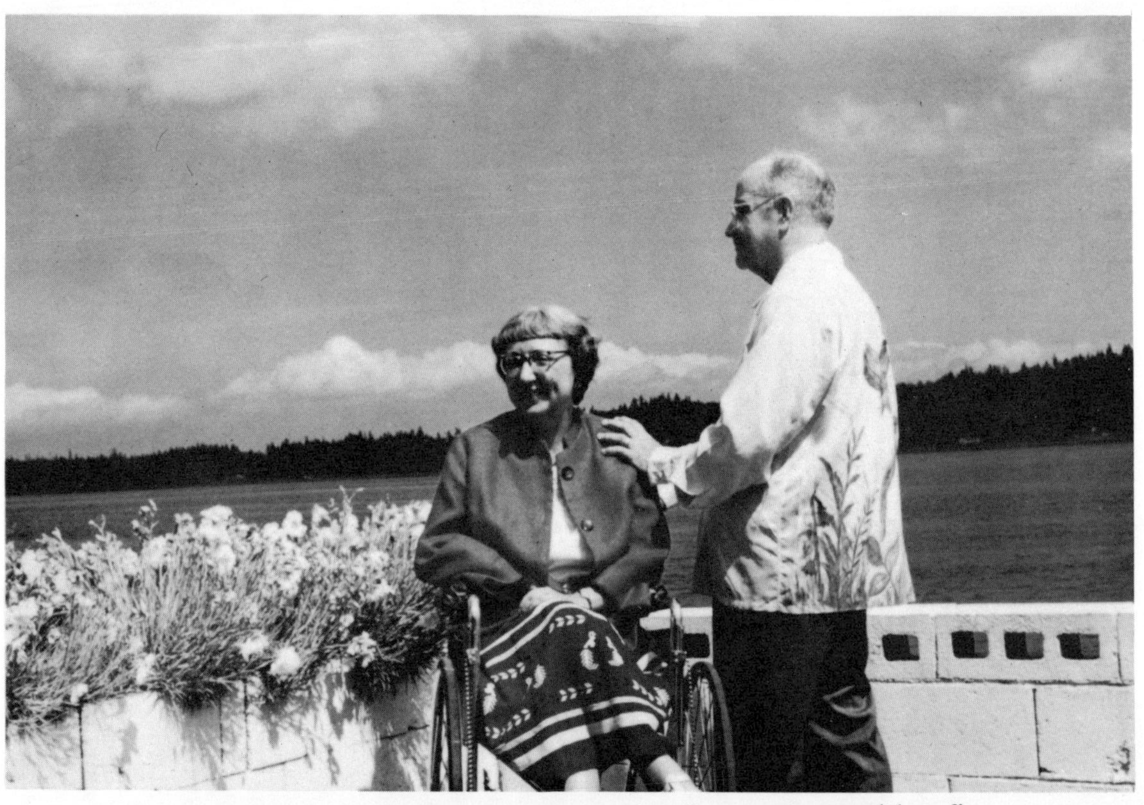

. . . a wheelchair marriage that brought happiness and mutual benefit pharmacy in Seattle. Before leaving in the morning, he set me up for painting tiles, something I had dreamed of doing for some time. With all my materials placed on my long work-table, I could wheel from one position to another, operating my chair by twitching my hips, since my hands were useless for moving the wheels.

A picture of a stained glass window, in *Life* magazine, showing a monk kneeling by a table pouring wine from a stone jar seemed an interesting subject, and led to a series of tiles on "Medieval Wine Makers." I began by making sketches of various orders of monks, vineyards, grapevines, burros and baskets. I kept the idea of stained glass windows by breaking up the background, drawing the outline on the tile with a wax marking pencil, then using black decal enamel for the outline of each section. Using only primary colors, I worked in small areas because the paint dried fast, got sticky and produced air bubbles if stirred, but it was fascinating. This type of enamel paint produced a glass-like effect.

To complete the series, I needed a picture of a wine press which I finally found on a twelfth century tapestry. Now it seemed inevitable that I make a large wall piece combining all the ideas into a single picture representing a stained glass window with an arched top. Because I was not able to reach out to paint, I did one tile at a time, occasionally placing two together to make the color continuous. The finished work was three (6 x 6 inch) tiles wide and eight tiles high. The central figure was a bishop blessing the vintage, around him monks carrying on the various activities involved in the process of harvesting grapes and making wine, with the castles and monastery on the hill in the distance. In the arch I put a stylized pattern of bunches of grapes. As I finished each tile, Frank arranged it with the others on the floor so that I could study the total effect. While the actual painting took only one hundred fifty hours, the research and sketching kept me occupied for several months. Mounted on one inch plywood, trimmed with a black line, the work became a sturdy and quite effective wall panel. "Medieval Vintage" was followed by a monastery garden scene which my brother, Charles, bought for a coffee-table top, and led to another series on the "Windows of Chartres." Frank put each tile, on completion, into the oven to set the protective clear enamel recommended to make the glazes more durable.

These projects brought to an end my "adventure in art." One afternoon I knocked over a jar of enamel. Trying to set it up, I spilled another. It was then I realized that dystrophy was again on the move, involving muscles used in reaching out.

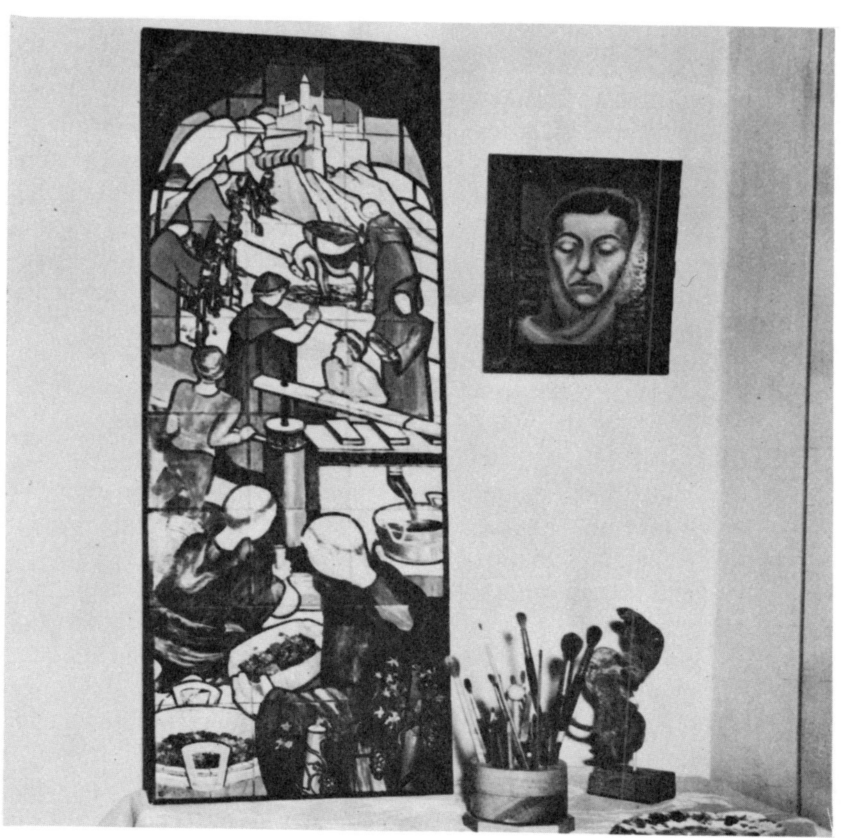

Before leaving in the morning, Frank set me up for painting tiles.

Chapter 7

CRISSCROSSING CALIFORNIA

To counteract the discouragement of this new limitation, Frank insisted on a short vacation. He packed me in the car and headed for California. Wheels on wheels, we traveled down the Oregon coast, a thrilling experience with its beautiful, surging ocean seen for miles from the car. Motels on the water's edge provided views from the picture windows. We visited the Redwoods, memorable for the beautiful trees with light shimmering through.

This trip, and those to follow, have convinced me that all disable-bodied spirits should take to the open road if they can possibly do so. Traveling today is easier for the physically handicapped than many realize. Our superhighways cut through areas of beauty and grandeur which can be enjoyed without leaving the car. Service stations with their easily accessible rest rooms are located everywhere.

Modern motels where Frank and I stayed were warm and comfortable—often more luxurious than many of our homes. These motels usually have few or no steps at all and cars can be driven up to the door for unloading "the patient." There is usually a restaurant nearby for late dinners and early breakfasts.

Of course, Frank saw to it that I was comfortable in the car. He had a foam rubber footrest attached below the dashboard so my feet could be stretched out part of each day; a sturdy wedge pillow made for my back; and of course the safety strap designed especially for me by Frank. I carried a tray that snaps on my wheelchair in case restaurant tables were too low to slip my chair beneath.

In San Francisco, we went to Fleishacker Zoo. We took a

safari through the Natural History Room. We found many places that can be visited "by wheelchair"—the Aquarium, Chinatown and even Fisherman's Wharf.

After short visits with wonderful friends, we started home through San Francisco, over the Golden Gate Bridge, to Highway No. 1, a little-traveled road along the edge of the ocean, with sheer cliffs below at the left and mountains to the right. Suddenly we came upon a clearing with several historic buildings. It was Fort Ross, a settlement made by the Russians in 1812. They had come to seek otter hides. The blockhouse, stockade and cannons, the curator explained, were to protect the Russians from the Spaniards!

I was interested in the church, which was of early Russian architecture, and made a watercolor sketch which I added to others made along the way—the Church of the Wayfarers in Carmel, the Danish Town of Solvang and San Francisco's Chinatown. Into each of these I drew line sketches of myself in the wheelchair in the foreground. I thought I could use them to illustrate an article that might inspire others who are handicapped to travel. I did send them to a couple of national magazines, but they came flying back to me. These little sketches were done with the last of my painting strength. I knew I would have to fill the time with a new interest. But at least I could hope that the "art period" had given me a good foundation for whatever I might pursue.

Chapter 8

THE INDOOR SPORTS CLUB FILLS A VOID

For several years I had been urged to join an organization for handicaps called the Indoor Sports Club, but I resisted all invitations, because I felt I wanted to associate with only able-bodied people. I had the notion that my mind might weaken like my muscles if I didn't! I recognize this now as the denial often encountered in the physically handicapped who have not as yet adjusted to their condition and who do not want to be identified strongly with the thirty million or more in our country who are physically limited. This is one factor which continues to prevent the successful formation of a strong national lobby, a force greatly needed if uniform legislation and other advantages are to be gained.

Suffering from the void left in my life when painting became impossible, I at last accepted an invitation to the Indoor Sports Club's Thanksgiving dinner. About sixty handicapped members were seated at a long, narrow table being served by a group of volunteers. My main impression of the day was a feeling of being overwhelmed by so many others with physical disabilities. In my family circle, I had been the only unusual person. Here I was confronted with dozens of people who were more handicapped than myself. It was a traumatic experience. I thought of helping them, but they all seemed so self-reliant that I didn't feel needed.

Soon afterwards the Club took me to the Shrine Circus. It was a first for me. Led through the "Animal Entrance" on ground level, we found wheelchair space within a few feet of the lions' cage! The next week we were all guests at Seattle's "Aqua Follies" staged at Green Lake Amphitheatre. By now I felt this group might afford an outlet for my energies. I cast my lot with them, but it was at least a year before I felt confortable enough to speak up and offer to serve on a committee.

I finally became a crusader for clubs for the handicapped. When I say clubs, I mean groups organized by the handicapped for the handicapped. When a person has been disabled severely, his usual scope of activity is sharply reduced. Adjustment to the revisions in daily living become a difficult emotional experience. The hardest may be social readjustment.

The club offers social contacts and much more—a chance for active participation in the business and management of the club or in committee work; a chance to attend classes, taught by professionals in the fields of arts and crafts, writing, printing and music; and a chance to help fellow members, new ones in particular, to overcome the sense of being "out of things."

Chapter 9

WHEELS ON WHEELS THROUGH THE SOUTH

Frank had been quietly making plans for a motor trip through the South and into Mexico. It seemed incredible to me, but all things seemed possible to Frank. We were on the road November 20, 1952, enjoying the riot of autumn golds of the trees and shrubbery as we followed the coast road, which hangs to the cliffs above the ocean with an awe-inspiring tenacity, to central California. During the next five months, we covered ninety-five hundred miles across eight states and well into Mexico.

We stayed several weeks in Texas with my sister and her husband (the ones whom I had lived with in St. Louis). Then on to visit my nephew and his family in San Antonio, where I wheeled around the Alamo, the Spanish Governor's Palace, the San Jose Mission (to see its famous sculptured Rose Window), and La Villita, which is the little restored settlement in center city.

On a warm sunny morning in January, we took off for our New Orleans adventure. We approached New Orleans at sunset and I'll never forget the weird effects of the gnarled trees in bayous, their branches fringed with Spanish moss, silhouetted against a fiery red-orange sky. New Orleans—an exciting mixture of old and new, a city I never expected to see! In the French Quarter, we wandered through antique shops, peeked into the sunlit courtyards and feasted on superb Creole dishes served out-of-doors—all so easy for my wheelchair!

Our next stop was Liberty, Texas, near Houston, to visit the famed Woods Sisters, who put the first spotlight on our common disease. Nadine and Sallie Woods were stricken in childhood. After involving several doctors and promoting an MD Correspondence Club of over two thousand patient-members, they organized the National Muscular Dystrophy Research Foundation in 1950. At about the same time the New York-based Muscular Dystrophy Association of America which was so vigorously supported by a Dean Martin-Jerry Lewis Telethon in 1954, raised $5 million for MD research. Sallie and Nadine, vivacious and cordial, gave us a tour of their foundation headquarters, and renewed our vigor to create a major center for handicaps in Seattle.

Our long, warm winter in the South ended with a trip into Mexico as far as Monterey. There we found a city of contrasts—wealth and poverty, historic and ultra-modern architecture.

It was near Christmas and there was a fiesta-like feeling in the colorful shops. We wanted to take home everything in sight. For myself, I settled on a peasant blouse and full red skirt with a beautifully embroidered band.

Briefly, the trip home included Arizona's Petrified Forest, the Grand Canyon, Hoover Dam, and Las Vegas. As we approached Seattle we saw fresh green leaves and early flowers. We realized that we had seen Spring four times. As we had followed the sun south in November, so had we followed its northward journey in April; my wheelchair had kept pace with Old Sol!

Chapter 10

SEATTLE HANDICAPPED CENTER—A REALITY!

Big things had occurred within the Indoor Sports Club during the few months we were away. A publisher had joined our ranks as well as an insurance man who had been in political and labor union public relations before he was stricken with polio. The three of us became known as the "Triumvirate of Dreamer-Doers," and we did indeed lead the club into a grand new adventure.

The *Good Samaritan* had been established as a club publication which would tell the story of our activities and aims and, through advertisements, bring a regular income. Although the club provided transportation and I was not dependent upon Frank, he became intensely interested in our projects. I soon found that he was working as hard for the club as I.

One of our first services was to offer transportation which, I strongly feel, will be a perpetual problem until our society meets the need of transporting physically disabled people. I especially remember one Sunday when I rode with Frank to pick up club members. We stopped for an older member and I was horrified to see the long flight of outside steps, knowing that she would be on crutches. We went to another house where a member, crippled with arthritis, came up a flight of stairs from the basement. I knew she should not be living there. Such experiences—and there were many others—made me aware of the great need for an especially designed apartment for disabled adults. This would be the project I was determined to promote. The idea became reality in 1969 when Center Park Apartments for the Handicapped was completed. Its birth was not without pain. We had to strengthen

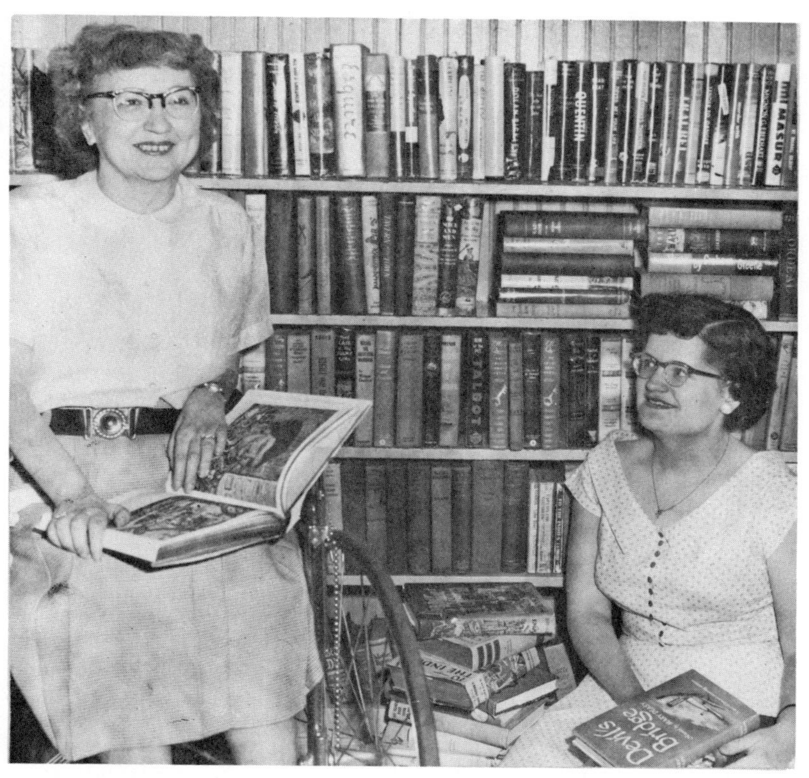

Handicapped members found it convenient to enter our house by ramp and get books from the library which I had established in an unused front room across the hall from our apartment.

the club, build its membership and convince the community and government of our need.

Club meetings had been held in the old Armory downtown. It was adequate in some ways, but newer members felt it cold and depressing. Frank secured the use of the new Junior YMCA recreation room in the University district for one Sunday each month. Located directly across the street from our apartment, members who came there for planned recreation found it convenient to enter our house by ramp and get books from the library which I had established in an unused front room across the hall. My niece, Judy, who lived upstairs, became the first librarian.

My first assignment as a member of the Indoor Sports Club, which later became the Seattle Handicapped Club, was in publicity. The chairman had asked for volunteers and I remarked that I could get an article in the *University District Herald* because a neighbor, who often helped me, was mother of the editor. The paper printed an article with a picture of us in my apartment. It included a plea for volunteers to help with transportation, food and entertainment.

I now had much phoning to do and soon realized that dialing with a stick in my mouth would cut down on my usefulness. I called the phone company and four engineers came to study my problem. The instrument they devised served perfectly for fifteen years. It allowed me to dial by operating a lever with my elbow, moving a needle indicator to the desired digit. A smaller key, operated by a downward pressure of my elbow, performed the equivalent of raising or replacing the receiver. A standard headset mounted on a flexible arm was conveniently adjusted so that I could roll up and place my head at the receiver. With this help I soon recruited a large group to help us.

Two years later I was installed as president of the club. One of my first acts was the setting up of a Building Committee to secure a site for a club building and promote its development. About this the board of directors had been in conflict, some

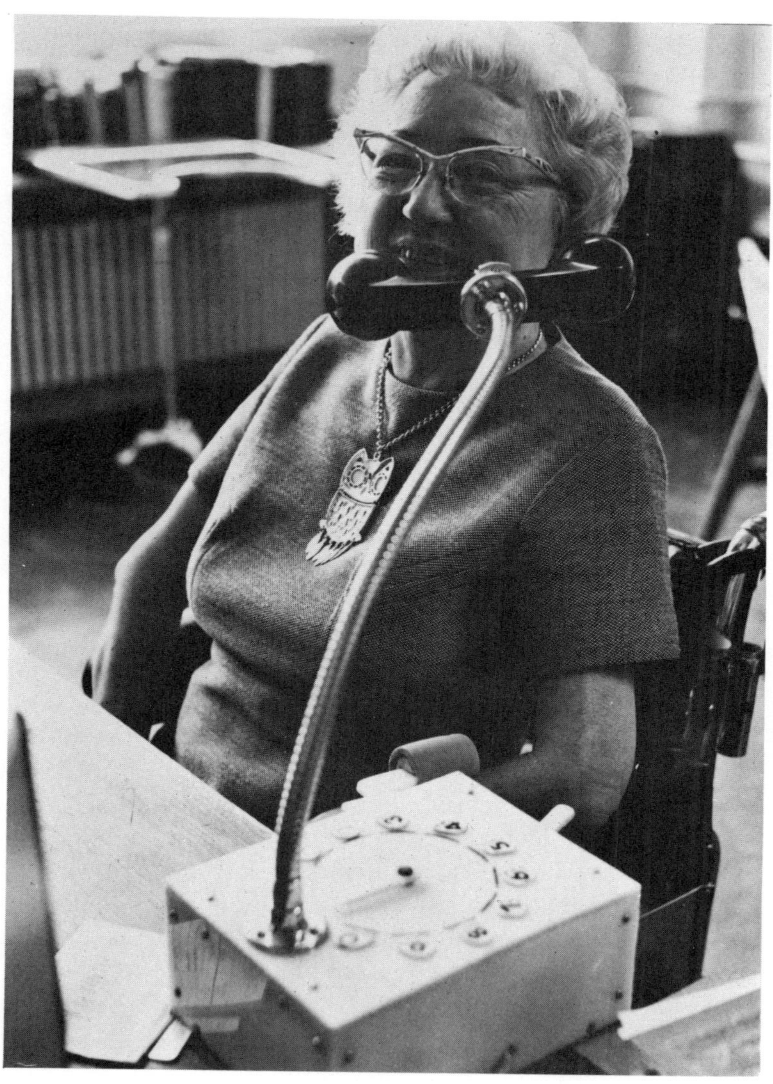

And here I am waiting for a phone call, maybe from you.

wishing to find a location immediately, while others felt the club was not ready for such a large undertaking. As president, I took the issue to the membership, presenting the need and the plans. The membership voted overwhelmingly for a Building Committee.

We hired a University of Washington research man to help us get community support. We knew our need but it was necessary to convince others. The survey found that an estimated ten thousand handicapped people lived in the area, and that the need for both more adequate housing and for a recreation center was acute.

We knew housing would have to wait for long-range planning, so we decided to establish the recreation center first. Each weekend the committee went out looking for land or buildings. A list of available buildings was secured from the mayor's office and the tax-title office. Inspecting the areas offered, we found they were in ravines, in undesirable locations or extremely high-priced. We were a bit discouraged, but one member suggested, "Let's try the Park Department."

We began attending the Park Department meetings. We made our wants known. Though they had no land or buildings, they were sympathetic to our plans. This contact led us to Federal Housing, which had listed two buildings in Rainer Valley. Frank and I drove down to look them over. I had received the key by mail. As we drove up, the police were right behind us and I was glad we had the letter and key in hand.

Later the committee joined us. The building was boarded up. We entered in pitch darkness, wheels and crutches crunching through broken glass. The place was desolate, filthy and depressing, but we knew immediately that it was the right size and in the right location.

Both the buildings were in a large, open area of several blocks covered with high grass. We often spoke of the area as our "cow pasture." Though we found the buildings in February, 1955, it was 1957 before all the complications of ownership were worked out between King County, the City of Seattle and the federal government. The buildings were then put under the jurisdiction of the City Park Department. The job of restoration was ours. We recruited carpenters, electricians, painters, cleaners, plumbers and ditch diggers who pitched in voluntarily to renew the first building we were to use. It had been heated by a coal furnace, so renovating meant installing an oil burner. We also had to bring a new water main from a meter a block away.

During the early days of reconstruction the club board of directors had a meeting in the building so that the members could see what was being done. The boards on the outside of window openings had not been removed, but we did have electric lights. During this meeting, one of the amputee members, a tall, strong man in spite of his disability, went to a window where people were trying to remove the boards. He raised his wooden leg, gave a huge lunge and the whole board popped off. We cheered at the first sight of daylight in our building.

Reconstruction was speeded up by plans to host a meeting of Northwest Handicapped Clubs. The ramp was in, the toilet room enlarged, new windows had been installed and painting was in progress; but we still had no tables. I heard about some that were being discarded at Smith Tower. They were for sale at one dollar each. Via "elbow" I negotiated by phone and got a volunteer trucking service to bring them to the Center. They were about thirty inches square and thirty inches high, a good height for wheelchairs. We secured 4 x 8 sheets of plywood, put them end-to-end between each set of tables and placed them down the length of the room. My niece, recently married, loaned us her new sheets, which were used for tablecloths. Along the side of the building there was a row of rose bushes, long neglected, but in full bloom. Frank picked small bouquets and placed them in water glasses the length of the table. It looked elegant to those of us who had seen the room at its worst!

Chapter 11

"LADY ON THE SPOT"

In September we had the formal dedication of the Seattle Handicapped Center. It was attended by city councilmen, county commissioners and members of the Park Board. "Our hope," I told the group, "is that this Center will be a beacon light that will draw all the handicapped people of this community for friendship and recreation."

Months before the Center opened, I had filled several pages of a planning notebook with possible activities. In fact, I had used it to show various officials how valuable a center for the handicapped could be. There was little available in the way of recreational opportunities at that time. Park Departments had not entered the field, and rest homes made little or no effort to provide such services. From my own experience, I realized the therapeutic effects of creative outlets, and added art and craft classes to the club program at once. Both were an immediate success. My former contacts in art were useful and soon I had recruited a loyal and experienced staff of teachers, helpers and new volunteer drivers.

I found one of my most valuable assistants in a swimming pool. Betty Marion appeared one Monday morning during the free swimming hour which our club co-sponsored with Muscular Dystrophy and Easter Seal. I told her about the Handicapped Center and invited her to visit. The measure of her interest and her vital personality were evident when she arrived promptly the next morning. To get there she had to take a bus, transfer downtown, and finally climb a two-and-a-half-block hill—all of this effort on crutches.

As she left classes that day, I asked her if she would like to participate. She said, "I'm not interested in joining a class, but I can teach almost anything." She began with a small group in wood mosaic, then she catalogued the growing library, and within a short time she was put on the staff as my assistant. With her talent, competence and love for people, she became invaluable. When she acquired a car with hand controls and a car-top lift, she and I began attending meetings of other organizations working with the disabled. It was the kind of communication we needed most.

Margaret Andreasson, the wife of one of the Club drivers, was my co-director at this time. She had been deeply involved in musical circles. The thought of helping us have a stronger crafts and music program occurred to her one day and she called me. She obtained a prominent voice teacher to lead a singing class; she arranged an appointment with a relative who had a pottery shop in her home and who, though crippled by arthritis, offered to teach ceramics and also to bring several of her students as assistants. A Lions Club provided a kiln and we launched the popular ceramics class, which has provided social and therapeutic enjoyment continuously. Many have exclaimed, like the cerebral palsied young man when his first piece was taken from the kiln, "Did *I* make *that*!"

We obtained instructors in weaving through Paul Brown, who was then the Park Department superintendent. He asked one day during a meeting at the Park Department if we planned to offer weaving, and I answered rather hesitantly, "If it is possible." Then he volunteered the help of his wife, Florence, who, he said proudly, "is one of the best weavers around here." She came with five women who had been weaving with her and they have been our instructors each Thursday afternoon for 14 years. We now have 16 looms.

As the word of the new center spread, we began to have visitors from medical schools, vocational rehabilitation, visiting nurse services, park departments, rest homes and many other agencies. Their enthusiasm convinced me that we had taken the right approach.

It was soon apparent that we must negotiate with the Park

Department for another building which stood nearby, boarded up and abandoned. Our maneuvering was a bit devious, but it worked. The head of our weaving section, whose husband was superintendent of Parks, suggested that we put all the looms together on dining room tables and invite someone from the park department to see our working conditions. When the park inspector walked in, his first words were, "My goodness, you are crowded! You certainly do need the other building!" So we began renovating, ramping and repair, and we named the new structure the Center Arts and Crafts Building. Our membership ranks soon grew to three hundred—one of the largest clubs solely organized and supported by handicaps in the country.

At this high point, my own life took a sad and tragic turn. Frank suffered a massive stroke and never lived to see the renovation of the second building or the completion of our great goal to house the handicapped in comfort. In trying to reconstruct my own life, I was faced not only with the loss of a loving companion and assistant, but my mobility was again a problem. I needed to be driven to the Center almost every day to keep it running smoothly.

My cousin, Clarice, who had come to stay with me part-time, was not strong enough to care for me. One day it came to my mind that if I left my apartment, she could stay and be the manager. So I called the committee and applied for the job of "resident janitor" in the new building!

Two months after I lost Frank, I moved into the building. While I was attending a district meeting in Salem, Oregon, my sisters, assisted by the fireman in charge of our Muscular Dystrophy swim hour, moved the essential belongings from my apartment to quarters in the new building. When I returned, I came to the Handicapped Center instead of going home. This made the transition easier. Here I had only to wheel from my bed-living room to my office. I literally immersed myself in developing the building and expanding the programs, leaving no time for personal grief.

So I became the "lady on the spot." The change was good for me and essential to the Center. It provided a permanent resident who could turn on the heat, lock and unlock doors, answer the telephone, direct workmen and janitorial help, order and receive supplies, guard against vandalism and alert the proper people in emergencies. The lady who cared for me and I were there at all times to welcome visitors and interview prospective members and volunteers.

Although I had been unable for several years to paint, the early drip paintings carrying "raves" in my art magazine prompted me to brazenly remark that I could do as well by spreading a large canvas out on the parking lot and running over it with my wheelchair! A painter friend heard me and did not forget. She arrived early one Sunday morning with three big sheets of masonite and said, "Come on out here. You said you wanted to do it, and now is your chance."

In the past, I had noticed that on the papers dropped by my worktable, the swirls made by my front wheels were pleasing in design, and that the large back wheels made a complementary "rhythm." So, with the tires protected by masking tape, I ventured outside. Mrs. Howie had pre-painted the backgrounds and asked what colors I wanted to use and where I wanted them placed. She then put large daubs of paint on the backgrounds. I circled through them, spreading and mixing the colors as I turned. When we set them up in the storage room to dry, I was reluctant to let anyone see them. But a reporter who came to interview a visiting speaker, spotted them and insisted that we let him photograph them. They were even photographed for posterity with the governor of Washington!

The Center soon assumed a home-like atmosphere. Paintings by the art classes were on the walls. Cabinets held an array of interesting crafts. Voices and laughter permeated the rooms, Creativity, enjoyment, self-confidence and social adjustment were the gratifying results which drivers, teachers and helpers observed with a feeling of accomplishment. The center was my home for the next eleven years.

Much of our energy was directed toward our future goal—the building of Center Park Apartments for the Handicapped. We would have to raise funds and build community support. But this time we had experience, a growing membership, and a need that local and national government officials could not ignore.

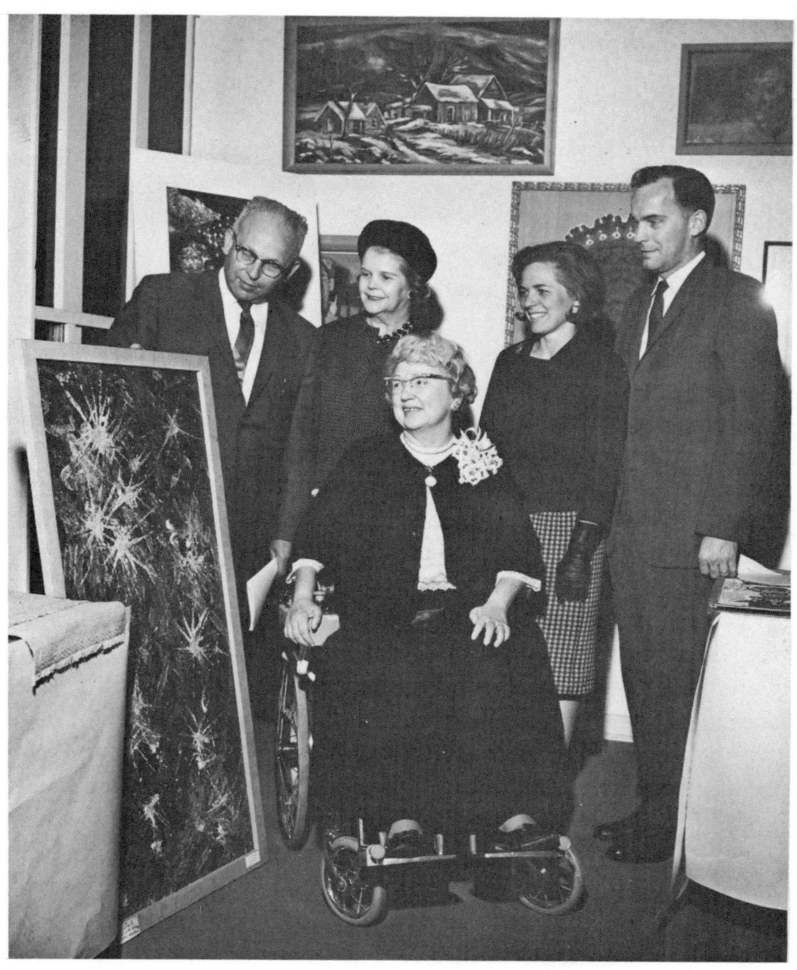

Governor and Mrs. Dan Evans and Mayor and Mrs. Dorm Braman join me in (I hope) amusement over my wheelchair's original oil. . . . All I did was steer.

Chapter 12

WINGS ON WHEELS—EUROPE

Because my youngest sister, Marion Hunter, graciously agreed to be my companion, I was able to accept the invitation to head the first "Wings on Wheels" tour of Western Europe, under the People-to-People Program inaugurated by President Eisenhower. We were "Ambassadors of Good Will," going to meet our counterparts in other countries. For thirty years I had been on wheels, so this was truly a great adventure. Five nurses accompanied the group as well as my sister. The airline provided us with narrow chairs for use inside the plane, and in Washington, D.C., we were transported from plane to plane in a portable lounge!

We visited Holland, Denmark, Switzerland, France and England. The red carpet was out for us in each country. We were taken to the beautiful and interesting places which tourists usually enjoy, and also to housing projects, schools, and rehabilitation sections of hospitals. We were shown one area in which a village was to be built for the handicapped. This was Het Dorp in Holland, near Arnheim. It has since been completed, and others are being developed in several places there.

Because of our own prospective plans for residence apartments for the handicapped, I wanted especially to visit the Hans Knudsen Platz in Copenhagen. It was the high point of the European tour for me. The collective flats were built by the Danish Society of Cripples (which numbered 3,000 handicapped persons at the time we were there). The advanced design and innovative features gave me many ideas for our future project. They had 170 apartments in the 11-story building, which also contained a complete respo (respirator polio) infirmary on the top floor and a workshop in the basement level. Here one could find housing, treatment, training, recreation, and even employment. Ample space was also provided for members of the family. In Denmark, it seemed the determined purpose of state and private agencies to keep families together and to restore the handicapped to a productive life—no one was to be left to deteriorate in idleness.

Our plane was late en route to Zurich and we missed our train. Nothing could have been more fortunate because it resulted in our continuing by automobile, which is the best way to see that enchanting country. The drive to Interlaken, where we were to rest for two days, took us along Lake Lucerne.

From Geneva, we flew to Paris where my sister and I skipped the organized sight-seeing to have a longer time for Notre Dame Cathedral and the Louvre. Later we attended a party arranged for our group at St. Cloud's Hospital by the young people who were interested in hearing about Seattle's Handicapped Club.

England was the last country visited by the "Wings on Wheels" tour of Western Europe. Our good luck with the weather accompanied us and we were able to see clearly the beauty of the countryside, and the complexity of London and its environs. Outstanding in England was our visit to the Spinal Injuries Center at Stokes-Mandeville Hospital, noted for its excellent rehabilitation program. Our sixteen-hour flight home proved to us and to others that the handicapped have endurance equal to the able-bodied traveler.

When we stayed overnight for a State Department briefing en route to Europe, it marked the second time Marion had been with me in Washington. On another occasion, I was there to do a little lobbying. The nation's capital is hardly designed to make the handicapped a happy tourist. I pointed out to congressmen and Federal officials with whom I had made appointments that, among other inconveniences, I could not drink from most of the water fountains because they were too high; I could not negotiate the wheelchair through restaurant aisles in public buildings; my wheelchair could not even go through most of the public restroom doors. Even with Marion, who describes herself as "part of my equipment," I could not overcome such barriers.

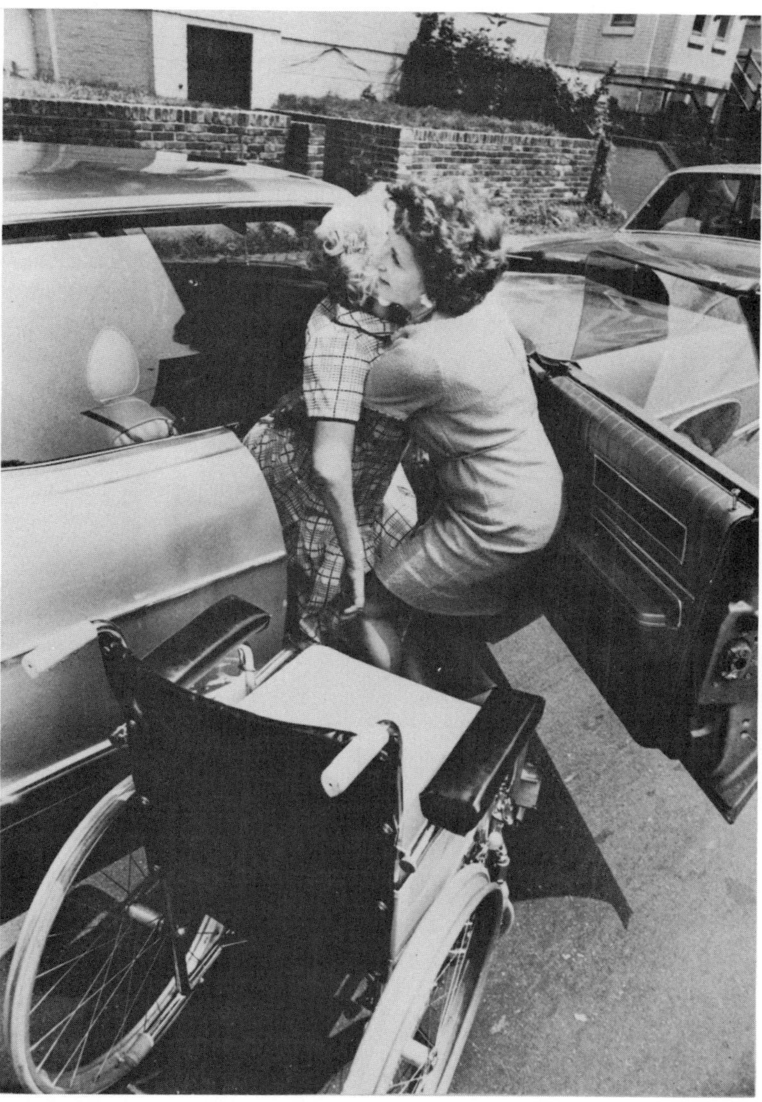

Even with my sister, Marion, who describes herself as "part of my equipment," I could not overcome some of the barriers in Washington, D.C.

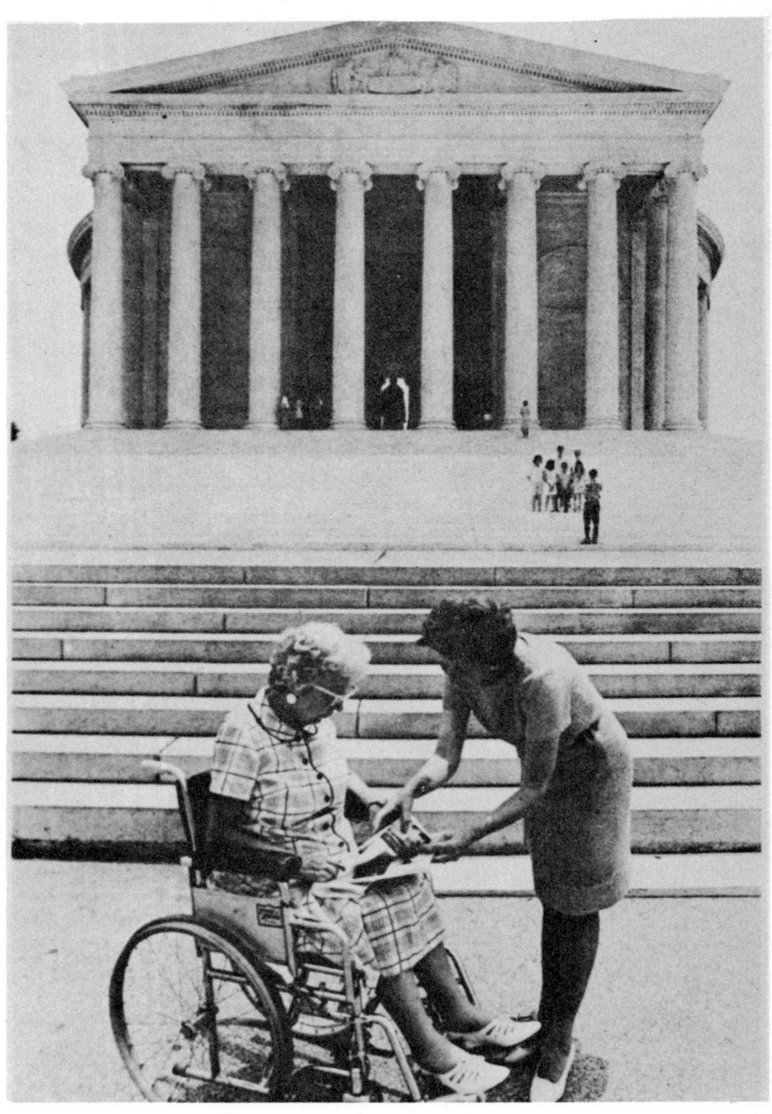

Sightseeing in Washington, D.C., leaves much to be desired for the handicapped, so I spent my time there lobbying against the barriers.

Chapter 13

DREAMER-DOERS!

By now ten successful, happy years at the Seattle Handicapped Center were behind us. We had every reason to believe that we had achieved the faith of the community in the ability of the handicapped to organize and implement our dreams. The next goal was housing of the handicapped in apartments designed especially for their convenience and comfort. Because this dream produced the first apartment building especially planned and built for the handicapped in the United States, a brief outline of how it was accomplished might serve as a plan for other communities.

The Building Committee compiled a list of fifteen names of people from the mayor's office, Welfare and Public Housing, private housing and every agency working with the handicapped, to act as an advisory committee. I did the telephoning, for I knew they were busy people who would be hard to contact. I expected excuses and rejections of our invitation for a meeting. To my amazement, not one single person refused. The whole concept was presented to them—a complex on this very site which would include not only the apartment building, but another structure which would house vocational rehabilitation, some therapy and a recreation social center replacing our present Handicapped Center. There was genuine enthusiasm. They suggested that we meet again soon to discuss ways of financing the project. We took our problem to the Seattle Housing Authority. The executive director had been with us in spirit since the day he turned over the key to the old building to us. At this second meeting he said, "If you are willing to go through with this stupendous adventure, I will carry the ball for you."

We agreed that nothing would be too hard and he took on the assignment, making application to the Federal Housing Administration. In Washington, D.C., the concept met with general approval. The Seattle Housing Authority received $27,000 for a preliminary survey. The figures from our former statewide survey were included in the report and the F.H.A. allocated $2.5 million for the construction of 150 specialized living units.

The first meetings of our Building Committee, with the executive director of the Seattle Housing Authority and the architects, were devoted to location and type of building. The land was already available—*our site*, which meant that our Handicapped Center would be razed.

The concept proposed for the apartment building was a high-rise with floors laid out in the shape of a cross, so that no one would have to go far to reach the elevator. Eliminating many of the prevailing architectural barriers, such as narrow doors and steps, we proposed a few special features to give maximum independence to the prospective residents. When plans were well advanced, a model walk-in kitchen and bathroom were built into our center for criticism and comment. This was helpful and prevented several serious mistakes.

We held a festive tenth anniversary celebration in September, 1967 to thank the scores of people who had supported us through those pioneering years. A few months later, we were given the deadline for evacuating the buildings. This stupendous undertaking was accomplished with the help of volunteers and donated trucks. The club offices and crafts were moved to a converted factory building near Lake Union. The contents of our two buildings had to be maneuvered into a single room forty-five feet square. We put each class in a corner with shelf space around it. The work tables, placed down the center, could be used alternately or in compatible combinations. We joked about being next door to a community psychiatric clinic, saying the crowding and confusion would send us there in no time, but to our gratification, there was no controversy or unpleasant situation in the three years we were there.

My own furniture and personal effects were moved at the same time. Since there was no living space in the temporary center, I went back to my former apartment building in the University district. I had wished to live near the newly located Center, but found it not feasible.

The University district, I found, was vastly changed from the quiet area that Frank and I had enjoyed, to a noisy hub of all that goes with modern youth and the protest movement. The change from my bucolic cow pasture to this noisy corner was most difficult. I gave up trying to sleep until after two o'clock when the drive-in nearby closed. I had thought to enjoy University Way again, expecting to go in and out of the fascinating shops independently, and alone, in my electric wheelchair. To my disappointment, all the driveways had been finished off with an inch or more rise so that my wheelchair could not negotiate them. The frustration would have pushed me into a protest march if one had come along. An article which I had written some time before titled, "Barriers Beware!" had been published in *Puget Soundings* magazine. We had won legislative battles requiring the removal of these barriers in new public buildings; but street curbs in Seattle had been our Waterloo. At about this time, it was my good fortune to be remembered in the will of a cousin. The money was promptly used for a van-truck (a la "Ironsides") with side opening and ramp to accommodate entrance of wheelchairs. This enabled me to go back and forth to the temporary club building for craft classes and to furnish transportation to others. Friends called it the "Ida Daly Special."

Finding someone to be the driver every day was a problem. I learned what it is to be dependent on neighbors and friends for transportation. One has to be strongly motivated toward getting out, because asking for help is not easy. Fortunately, a discerning young woman who lived next door volunteered to take me to Center classes. On days when I did not go to the Center, I began organizing a club auxiliary (using the telephone as my means of communication), helped coordinate transportation for others, and wrote for the club paper.

The paper was my pet project. I wrote almost all of the articles and news items (and still do many in current issues). How did I manage to produce typed copy for our paper? I just flipped my flippers! The idea for my "flippers" dates back to one time when I was being evaluated for the MDAA chapter. A therapist at the hospital fitted my chair with a pair of ball bearing "feeders" and set a dish of slippery canned peaches before me. I spent at least an hour trying to maneuver a slice on to the attached spoon and into my mouth. Finally the no-doubt-weary nurse said, "Mrs. Daly, I think you do much better by yourself without aids. Just keep on using both hands." I agreed, but the test had given me a feeling that perhaps I might paint or even type with such a device.

Some time later, I had an opportunity to test the idea. It became necessary for me to sit on a four-inch foam cushion, causing my whole orientation to my environment to be thrown out of focus. I was too high above all my tables, phones, washbasins, to function well. Finally I consented to put myself under the observation and testing of a team from the University of Washington's School of Rehabilitation Medicine.

The occupational therapist followed me around the handicapped center, measuring and testing whenever she could get me to sit still long enough. In the end, I was most grateful, because I am still using the built-up table tray and the "flippers" which she devised for typing. Up until that time, a stick, held in my teeth was my only means of using the typewriter. My arms make much better typists than my teeth!

The device is designed from the ball bearing arm supports which were constructed for polio patients and other quads. They consist of a metal tube which attaches to the frame of the wheelchair at the back. Into this, the jointed "arm" fits loosely so it swings freely, with little strength needed to move it backwards and forwards. At the end, toward the front, a sling of firm leather holds the arm from palm to elbow. There is a round metal plate lined with leather which braces the elbow and usually a spoon or pen is fastened to one's hand with a velcro band. The variation for typing, which was devised for me, consists of a metal strip extending from under my palm and projecting about three inches beyond the edge of the sling. To this is attached a metal tube about four inches long pointing downward toward the keyboard. It has a rubber tip which prevents slipping off the keys. I sit on an extra pillow, well above the table level and, using a device on each arm, I can reach all keys and controls. Of course, I need help in putting paper in the typewriter, but once set up, I can write quite easily and fairly rapidly, without tiring.

Since communication is one of life's greatest escape valves, this way of putting my thoughts down has been a great pleasure to me. It is much easier for a secretary to copy my typing than my handwriting and I do preparatory material for the Club publications, articles and rough drafts for letters. Since I use an old IBM billing machine, which is all upper case, and do not even attempt perfect execution, all of my writing except family letters are retyped for me. I feel like I am typing sixty words a minute as I speed along, only to find that I have spent thirty minutes on one page. I know this is a delusion, but it's a happy one!

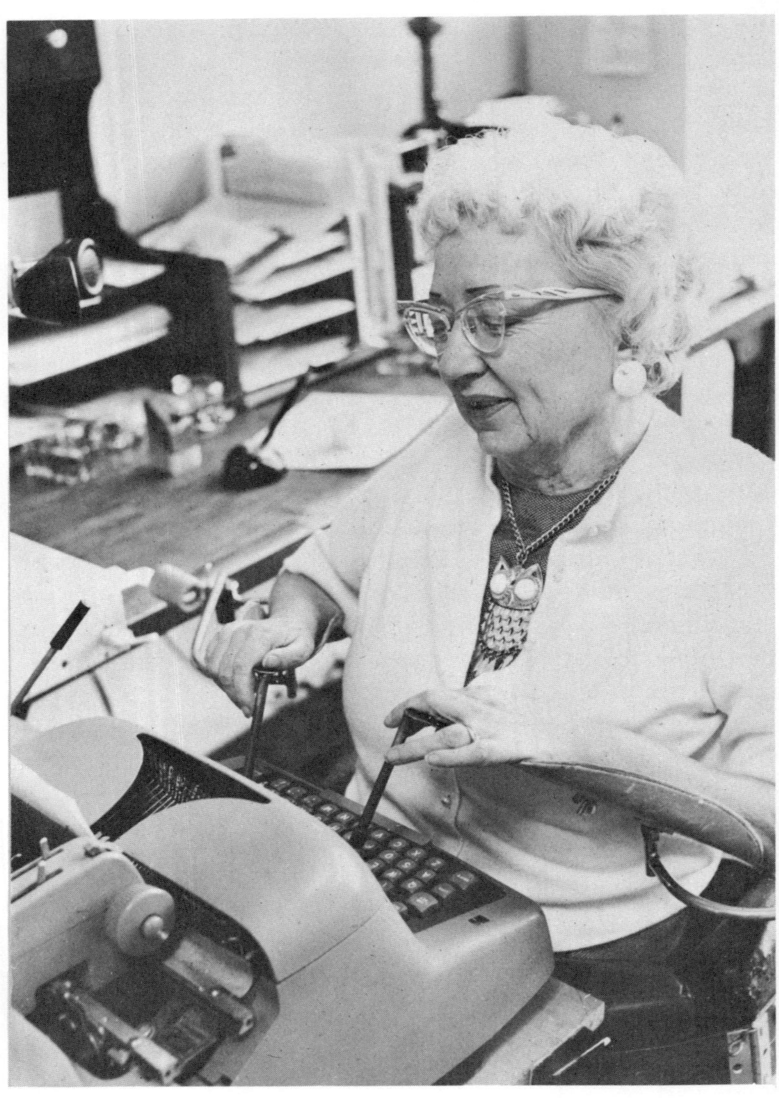

When I'm "flipping my flippers," my arms rest in the carriers and with my shoulder muscles I move the pegs over the keys to be punched.

Chapter 14

WHEELS ON WHEELS—CROSS-COUNTRY

When Betty Marion and I set out across the country one summer with a Congress of Organizations of the Physically Handicapped in Minneapolis as our "working" objective and New York as our "playing" objective, our qualms about tackling the trip were carefully masked. Friends and relatives were outspoken enough in disapproval. That we should face a cross-country trip by automobile, with nothing but nerve and the use of a few back, neck and arm muscles between us, appalled them. However, Betty's degree of paralysis from a spinal injury was comparatively slight. With crutches and short braces, she found few architectural barriers insurmountable and could drive, thanks to hand controls. Frankly, there were so many unanswerable questions that we decided not to plan any details of the trip beyond the bare skeleton of the itinerary.

Phyllis, who had moved across Puget Sound when her husband returned from duty in the South Pacific, eagerly consented to join us, although it meant lifting me many times a day and handling the luggage and wheelchair. Each day presented pleasures and problems, the latter being met with whatever degree of sportsmanship and good humor which we could collectively muster at the moment.

The Conference launched another effort to unite all clubs for the disabled: The National Congress of Organization of the Physically Handicapped. We enjoyed meeting workers from the East and Midwest. When State Councils of C.O.P.H. were authorized, I organized the Washington Council.

By now we were seasoned travelers in our own way and ready to go on to New York, where friends took us under their wings for a few days. Here especially we realized the comfort of credit cards (telephone and gasoline) as well as our Washington parking decal, which was respected out of state and which allowed us to use space in loading and theatre zones—all a boon in strange territory. We were especially grateful for the parking permit on the day that we barely made it to Manhattan for a matinee of *West Side Story*, after an inspiring visit at "Abilities Incorporated" on Long Island.

On the return trip we stopped at Cleveland to see the all-handicapped art show at nearby Chagrin Falls. The three hundred paintings had been done by mouth stick, toes, head or various combinations of the artists' remaining abilities. We also met those dedicated respos who had developed, with equally dedicated able-bodied friends, one of the most useful magazines in the field, the *Toomey J. Gazette*. The Chicago stop was social, visiting friends. In Montana, we circled down into Yellowstone and then sped home. We had enjoyed each other thoroughly and were not only still on speaking terms, but we were better friends than ever. We agreed that there are only three necessities for the handicapped traveler: the desire to get out and see the world; the adaptability to endure less than optimum conditions; and the ability to laugh at the incongruities which are bound to arise.

Chapter 15

CENTER PARK RISES!

After ground breaking on May 1, 1968, Center Park Apartments rose steadily into the air to become a seven-story, beautifully constructed high-rise for the handicapped, the first of its kind in this country.

Center Park is a handsome, modern building of red brick, masonry block and concrete. Most of the 150 units for the low-income disabled have one bedroom. There are a few two-bedroom units and a few efficiencies. Actually, the per unit cost of the building was only a little more than standard design, but the value to the tenants cannot be measured in dollars. Income eligibility is the same as for any Seattle Housing Authority building—25 percent of income-less-10 percent, is the basis for rents; $300 a month is the income ceiling, and assets may be as high as $12,000. Special eligibility requirements were set by a committee formed by the Authority. The first to be accepted were those in wheelchairs, next, those wearing braces, using crutches, canes or having severe mobility limitations. The last were those who might be able to adjust to average housing, but whose life would be better in such an apartment. This would include epileptics, heart cases, the partially sighted, et cetera. This selectivity slowed down complete occupancy by many months, and the Seattle Housing Authority is to be commended for resisting any pressures to open the doors to non-handicapped elderly or others whose needs were not as great as those with physical disabilities.

While I was living at Center Park, I wrote the following description of the apartment and my responsibilities as a Management Aide:

One of the most unique features of the apartments is the kitchen counter. With the built-in sink at one end, range top at the other and the work space with drawers in the center, the whole assembly can be raised or lowered to accommodate the needs of the occupant. There is open knee space under sink and range top. The oven is portable on a rolling utility cart.

Each unit has a private bathroom with tub; a roll-in shower on each floor is used by those who prefer showers or find them easier to manage than tub baths. We were required to choose all of one installation or the other, and we chose tubs; but it is still a debatable question.

We had also been obliged to decide on whether all units should have kitchens. As our main objective was to provide an opportunity for independent living, we voted "yes" on this one. Many changes have been made in housing laws since our year of decisions, and there is now more latitude in design. An alarming increase in building costs also forced us to give up some ideas. The simple expedient of mail boxes low enough to be opened from a wheel chair and the placing of electrical outlets high enough not to require stooping has in some cases made the difference between dependence and independence.

The two electric-eye entrance doors are indispensable and give a feeling of freedom, especially to quads such as myself. Appreciated are the extra-wide doors and corridors. Other doors are, unfortunately, much too heavy and it is hoped this will someday be remedied. Interior doors are all sliding, a great space-saving factor as well as being easy to manipulate. Closets and cupboards are fitted with flexible loops big enough to be pulled with arm or wrist.

In addition to these features are the very large window-ledge planting boxes for gardening, indoor-outdoor lounges on each floor, and a very large sun deck over the parking facility, accessible for barbecues, wheelchair square dancing, sports and other activities. The handicapped here can enjoy each other at their own pace.

So distinctive is Center Park design-wise that architects tour the unique facility to study the "barrier free" architecture which has finally awakened the builders of the nation.

My personal life at Center Park is a gratifying experience. It is part of my responsibility to show the apartments to incoming residents. Their expressions of surprise and pleasure are a daily joy. Finding furniture and other household necessities for those coming from hospitals and rest homes is a stimulating challenge, and setting up a recreation program which had not been included in the budget taxed one's ingenuity. I have initiated a system of floor monitors; two residents in each wing who watch unobtrusively for signs of any illness or accident. If milk or papers are not taken inside an apartment as is customary, the monitor reports it to our office. A residents' council has been set up and a steering committee organized.

Activities initiated include weekly game nights, classes, trips and tours, outside entertainers, et cetera. A weekly grocery shopping car has been recruited and arrangements made for delivery to those not going out.

As an answer to residents' need for extra help in housekeeping, I have accepted an experimental training program for retarded girls. Under supervisors, they come in every morning at eight and work until one. Although this particular group is not entirely satisfactory to everyone, I believe that a mutual need for opportunity and help makes this combination potentially valuable in housing for the physically limited.

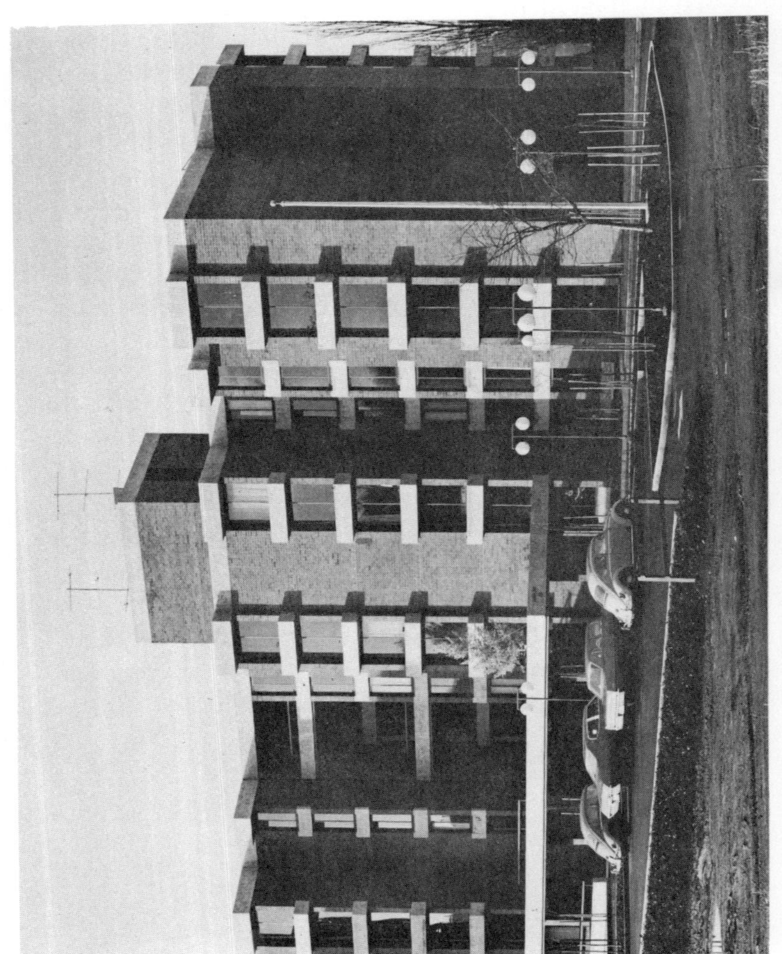

Center Park Rises!

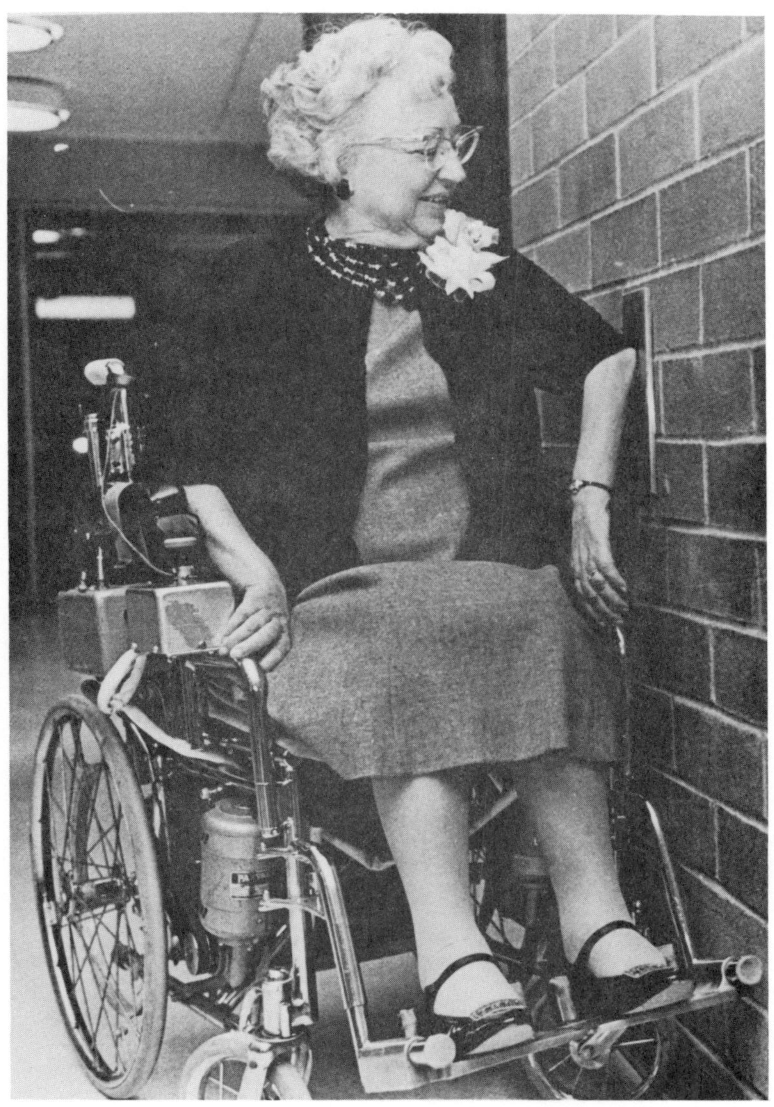

Elbows call elevators at Center Park.

Chapter 16

WINGS ON WHEELS—NEW YORK

One day when I was working at Center Park, a doctor came to my office with a question that opened an exciting vista. Could I and would I be available the next month to speak at the joint Convention of the American Academy of Physical Medicine and the American Congress of Rehabilitation Medicine? The meetings were to be at the New York Hilton Hotel. My inner response was a quick "yes," but my audible answer was more cautious. The trip would involve a replacement for my job and a traveling companion, which would double the expense. He quickly assured me that, since I was to be there by invitation, my expenses would be paid plus a hundred dollar honorarium.

The niece whom I have mentioned as the club's first librarian, had learned how to take care of me during those days and is still able to lift me without the mechanical aid which I have used since Frank died. She had flown to Texas with me, where we visited my nephew, Bob, and his family and wheeled around the spectacular Hemisfair in San Antonio. Now once more she arranged her family responsibilities and we again put wings under my chair.

Since we arrived at six in the morning, we saw New York asleep. The convention, which began that afternoon, was tremendous—exhibits including the most recent equipment and procedures in modern medicine.

My talk was part of a forum on "Creative Living: The Search for Adequate Housing after Rehabilitation." Of course, I was there to tell about "Center Park Apartments in Seattle, Washington." My topic was "A Public Housing Project for Handicapped Persons." Slides were shown emphasizing the architectural features that made living there convenient and pleasant. The question period brought out the doubts still in some minds regarding advisability of many handicapped people living in the same building. My contention was, and still is, that the advantages far outweigh the social worker's concept that this can be interpreted as "segregation." It was gratifying that my remarks and my report were reprinted in *Archives*, the official journal publication of the organization, with a photograph of Center Park Apartments.

At the close of the convention. my niece, Jean, and her husband urged me to come to Bryn Mawr, Pennsylvania, to tell the story of Center Park Apartments to a group on the Main Line trying to get a similar project underway in the greater Philadelphia area. They sent a car for us and the driver deposited us at their doorstep. They had arranged for me to see William Tubbs in Devon, who was gathering support for his "Faith Village" which would be designed along the lines of Het Dorp in the Netherlands. I gave my slide talk again and related the long years of effort that went before seeing our Center Park Apartment rise. I liked getting more mileage out of my speech as well as my wheelchair.

Chapter 17

THE "PLUS BUILDING"—THE SOUND OF HAMMERS

Upon my return to Center Park Apartments, I found that our Handicapped Club Board and the executive director were still struggling to work out finances for the rehabilitation-recreation building to replace ours, which had been razed to make way for the apartment. The story of frustration, road-blocks, and disappointments would fill another book. The government grant could not be accepted because of the terms included in its offer. Specifications put upon the building were so stringent that construction costs would be astronomical. The Club struggled through a maze of poor judgment, misguided information and bureaucracy for six months after the opening of Center Park Apartments. We finally had to admit that a new construction for the club adjacent to Center Park as planned would be delayed for many years if it depended on our Club's efforts alone.

About this time, the American Red Cross began construction of a new building, and their old location on Second Avenue was advertised at a price within our means. After many meetings and discussions with donors who pledged funds, a decision to buy the property was made.

It took a bit of daring to hold the annual meeting of the club during the first week while everything from the temporary center was being moved in. But everyone was eager to see the long-awaited *permanent* Club headquarters and did not worry about possible discomforts. We knew that it could not top the first day at the old quarters when the gas heaters didn't work and a snowstorm beat against the windows!

Our Club was now on the threshold of another adventure. This spacious, permanent brick building would house our present programs and expanded services, which we hoped to initiate. Our new tool for the implementation of these goals had already been developed by our Club, namely, The Northwest Institute for Rehabilitation and Research. It is, I believe, the first such institute founded by a group of physically handicapped persons.

Knowing that retirement age would soon end my work at Center Park, the board of directors asked me to again resume the responsibilities of executive director at our new headquarters. They built in an apartment for me on the second floor, reached by an elevator with a starter button just right for my elbow!

It was mid-March, 1971, when the Seattle Handicapped Club took possession of the building purchased from the American Red Cross. Wayne Clark, our treasurer and executive secretary, found a plush velvet red cross among the debris left behind. He took it home to his little daughter, Lisa. This knowledgeable "Treasurer's treasure" had learned her signs. "Look, daddy," she said, "it's a plus sign!" From then on we have always referred to the new Handicapped Center as the "Plus Building."

No designation could better describe the facility which resulted from the years of determined effort devoted to acquiring an adequate building for the Club. It has space, plus; it has location, plus; it has convenience, plus; and the potential which can best be symbolized by a quarter-turn of the plus sign to form an "X." We can now multiply many times the services and programs of the Club and its development arm, the Northwest Institute for Rehabilitation and Research.

Only Wayne's family and those of us who worked with him daily, can fully realize the extent of his sacrifice. Completely without self-interest, indifferent to physical weariness, ignoring mental strain, frustration, and repeated disappointment, he brought the Club to its objective. When the board of directors approved his decision to buy the building, he personally gained the consent of every donor group to change from proposed new construction to the available structure. Organization of the moving-in fell on Wayne's shoulders, as had the first move of the Center from South Hill Street to the Minor East location, in the spring of 1968 after ground breaking for Center Park Apartments.

The new building has more than twenty-five thousand square feet of space on two floors. Wayne covered every inch of it many times over as he planned alterations and supervised his incomparable crew of volunteers. Refusing the use of an electric wheelchair, he propelled his chair literally miles by arm-power and the use of his "good" leg. Since carpenters, electricians, plumbers and other volunteer workers often came after hours, he was at the Center days and evenings for many weeks. His enthusiasm was contagious and spurred us on.

His death came six weeks after the basic work was completed and the new Handicapped Center had been officially launched at dedication services. He had also arranged to reopen the supportive activities at the Fifth Avenue Hall and planned the annual Bazaar, which was headed toward a successful run with adequate space for every department, as we all had dreamed.

So it was with a mixture of emotions that I returned as Handicapped Center director—a feeling of great loss and at the same time a renewed determination to bring about the full potential of our new facility. Again, I was "on the spot," carrying out Wayne's plans with firms and volunteers until a new administrator could be named.

Enthusiasm has swept me along on every move the Club has made. We were now in the process of remodelling our fourth building. In between, we had watched with indescribable excitement and joy, the erection of Center Park Apartments for the Handicapped on the memory-filled site of our first remodelling venture. But this time there was a difference. The building we were developing was our own. So to enthusiasm was added the deep gratification that this would be a permanent location, adequate for the needs of the expanding programs we had always wanted to launch.

Part of the second floor of the Plus Building has become my home with living quarters, as well, for my housekeeper attendant. Ceiling-high windows of opaque glass run across the east walls of the entire apartment; one row of panes at eye level are of clear glass, affording a far view of the University district, a near view of many new office buildings, the Space Needle and the famous Washington Plaza Tower Hotel. The many attractions and cultural opportunities of Seattle Center, outgrowth of the 1962 World's Fair, are only a few blocks north. The business and shopping section of the city is nearby to the south. It is a fine location for Club-centered exploring and entertainment.

The street floor, accessible from a covered parking garage, as well as an electric automatic front door, houses the main offices, the craft class work tables, separate rooms for the kiln and ceramics supplies; our sixteen weaving looms; the library and music rooms (with a new Baldwin piano which my sister Hazel gave us) and a large open area for meetings, parties and the activities of special groups such as the Teens, Young Adults, and the Gavel Club. A large storage area has been transformed into a lapidary department and pottery studio. These two additions were made possible by a private gift from the daughters of our lapidary jeweler, James A. Boyle and grants from two local foundations, PONCHO and the Teachers' Foundation. These new creative crafts are especially designed for evening classes to serve the handicapped who are employed during the day.

An attractive gift shop and sales gallery, offering a wide variety of handcrafted items made by class members and units, faces the street. We also offer space to Seattle artists to display their paintings.

We encourage the handicapped to use the gallery as an outlet for the sale of their art and craft work. Many of them use their homes as studios and would not otherwise be able to

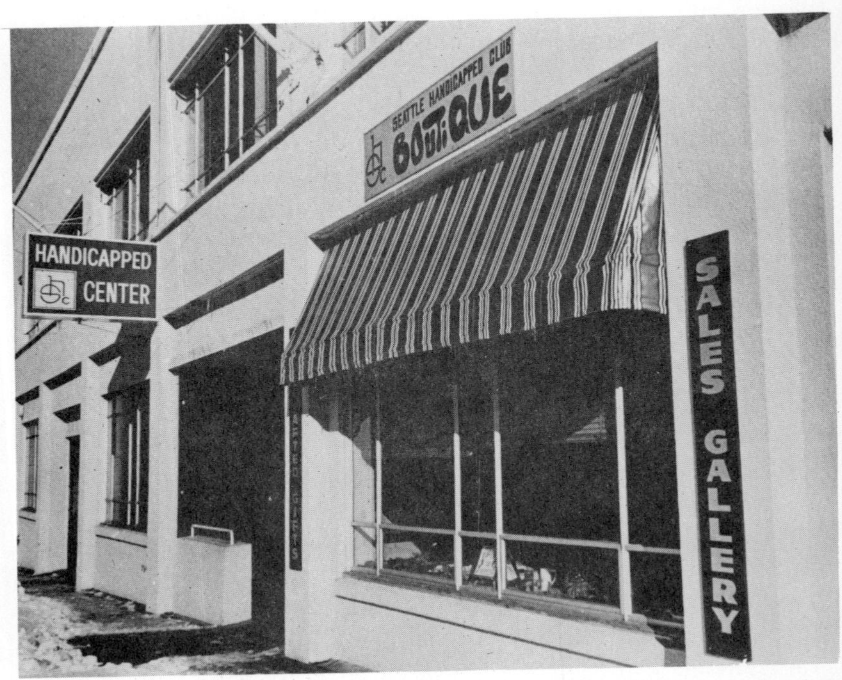

Our new permanent headquarters has an attractive gift shop and sales gallery, offering handcrafted items made by class members.

reach a market. I well remember how fast a home studio or workroom fills up. After all, there is a limit to how much one can store under the bed and behind the dresser!

Although there were members on the Club Board competent to fill the position of administrator, all had employment and family commitments making it impossible for them to give the time required. It was my first assistant director and New York travelling companion, Betty Marion, who suggested contacting a member who had shown interest in the Club through many years, although not participating actively in any of the programs. Kenneth Shellhase, a double amputee, had been understandably busy developing a home and farm, raising five children and working full time in agencies serving the physically and mentally handicapped. We approached him. The potential of our program seemed a challenge to him. Ken was hired as executive director of both the Club and its development arm, the Northwest Institute.

Our course is now set. At last we are implementing a long neglected plan to help the homebound. These members who never come to Club activities have been on my conscience for years. Now we will reach them with more than the monthly magazine and a few phone calls. I supplied our registered occupational therapist with a list of names of members who I felt would welcome such assistance. The first visits to the homes revealed what we had expected. The simplest devices, suggestions or information can make life unbelievably better—a lightweight reaching wand; velco on a checkers set; prismatic glasses; a ceiling-mounted interest board; a writing cylinder, mouth propelled; knobs on a typewriter carriage return. These are only a few results. We see this as a future project, to be funded as an employment opportunity service, as well as producing marketable and much needed aids for the disabled.

Our most recent help, in developing use of the second floor, came during the MDAA Western Section meeting in Seattle, when I was given a check to finance the large elevator required for several wheel chairs to reach the upper floor. The grant, authorized by New York Director Robert Ross and the Muscular Dystrophy board of directors, enables our center to operate at full potential. In England it would be called a "lift" which seems to me to be a symbolic designation. The second floor had remained an unknown area to most of the disabled because no activities could be held there. With the spacious new installation, five persons in wheelchairs and several standing can be carried at one time. It is, indeed, a "lift to life" for most of us. We are deeply grateful.

We have also acquired a new van with an electric loading platform. Its first trip brought wheelchair-bound young people to weekly craft classes from a convalescent home where most residents are elderly, affording them little companionship. These girls and others can now be brought in to young adult meetings and other club programs.

A generous grant from the Boeing Employees United Fund has provided an offset press and photographic equipment which expands our printing department, not only as a source of future revenue but as a training facility for the handicapped.

Center Park Apartments and the present Seattle Handicapped Center, once only dreams, are now realities. The handicapped will have them "for keeps," assuring their greater happiness and self-development in all the years to come. My story cannot be a personal biography. The past twenty years have woven the Handicapped Club and its projects inextricably together with the warp and woof of my own life. If the result can be in any way a pattern for future improvement in conditions for handicapped citizens everywhere—and there are thirty million of us—I shall be grateful.

Chapter 18

A PHILOSOPHY TO CHALLENGE DEPRESSION

Mention has been made of the black pall of gloom which clouded my childhood following several mishaps. Such periods of depression have not been frequent in my later life, but they did occur each time the advance of dystrophy forced me to give up an activity—first school, then walking, and then painting, with minor defeats interspersed along the way.

Gradually, I developed my own philosophy for climbing out of the pit. Gloom is boredom, I would tell myself over and over again. To escape, I sought some new interest within my remaining abilities. One time I even took voice lessons. It was one of my darkest periods and, although I am not particularly musical and no one ever told me I could sing, I found a private teacher who would work with me.

At other times, I would try a little self-analysis and offer myself some alternatives to recovery. I would say to myself, "If you remain negative, depressed and unmotivated, you will become immobile and probably bedridden in a rest home." That would scare me out of my wits *and* my depression!

A visiting lecturer gave me still another approach—gratitude. When life seems overwhelmingly dark, she said, begin to look around for things you still have and appreciate, no matter how small. Perhaps the artist in me made this approach work, for I could always find something of beauty in our natural surroundings, a flower, a bird, or a friendly smile.

But I feel sure the best philosophy, the one that has helped the most and requires no medication, is to stop thinking of one's self and concentrate on the needs of others. This effort flung me headlong into a life so full that there has been no time for personal emotional binges.

This formula has worked for me and countless others. So many of my colleagues at the Handicapped Center are outgoing, useful people. One of the best examples is Vincent Nordahl, who is perhaps the most physically handicapped person in our ranks. His excellent mind and fine artistic talents have found a valued outlet at the Center for fifteen years. (He illustrated the jacket of this book.)

Vincent's body is wasted and misshapened by the ravages of muscular dystrophy. The only remaining strength is a slight use of a finger and thumb of one hand. Yet he teaches a popular class in mosaics. He has been chairman of the board and, as head of the legislative committee, he has initiated and secured passage of bills which aid the handicapped throughout the state. He arranges Club theater parties and, in fact, acts in our own productions. My sister, Hazel, once visited when he was on stage playing a lead and she could not believe how the strength of his voice made her oblivious to his physical disabilities. At home, Vincent has built and operates a ham radio. He secures talent for our monthly socials and handles many matters for us on his special phone, designed with the help of a retired telephone company technician. I have never known him to be depressed.

Looking back, I believe I was more often puzzled than depressed over my illness. The sudden bursts of strength which surged through my body giving me false hope seemed inexplicable. How was it possible for muscles in arms, hands and legs to be weak one day and then strong enough the next to enable me to climb a hill behind our fruit ranch easily and then run home? This strange surging and ebbing of strength occurred many times during my earlier years, as has been related. No doctor could explain it. Muscular dystrophy was seen then as a progressive wasting of the muscles, which, unlike multiple schlerosis, did not involve the nerves.

Research at the Institute for Muscle Diseases, established by the National Muscular Dystrophy Assocation of America, and in other laboratories around the world, began in the

1960s to reveal many divergencies. Today it is known that there are a dozen or more types and combinations of symptoms. Patients are being re-tested and re-evaluated.

Although aware of this, I had resisted the suggestion of my friend, Kay Plumb, who is patient service coordinator in the Seattle MDAA office, to have another evaluation of my disability. After all, I insisted, what difference does it make now that I'm in my seventies to know what caused my ups and downs so many years ago. But I finally agreed to enter the MDAA clinic established by the King County Chapter at the University of Washington Hospital.

Both my history of strength lapses and the new tests indicated that I have had recurrent polyneuropathy, a secondary muscular disease or muscle atrophy which is caused by a primary nerve problem. The doctors said it would be impossible to put a name on the disorder without further tests which we both felt would be of little use to me or to science at this time. The new diagnosis gives a rational explanation of the physical basis of the swift changes I have experienced. It indicates that the defect lies in the nerve supply to the muscle or to the function between nerve and muscle fiber. Emotional, mental or physical states could have influenced the electrical impulses which in turn release chemical substances that initiate response in the muscle fiber. Research continues, but the present knowledge unveils partially at least my puzzling mystery.

We all have our own ways to keep up our spirits. Activity and involvement work for most of us. I believe my pioneering father gave me an extra dose of his own indomitable spirit. He would say, on a morning after a killing frost wiped out his entire fruit crop, "Oh, well, it's only ten months until the trees will be in bloom again!"

ACKNOWLEDGEMENTS

Although the original, motivating force came from the physically disabled themselves, development of the Handicapped Center and Center Park Apartments would have remained a nebulous, unrealized dream without the help of a few perceptive individuals at critical points along the way. One of the first of these was *Charles C. Ross*, executive director of the Seattle Housing Authority. As an invited guest at an early meeting of the Club's Building Committee, he listened to our plans and became convinced of our competence. The first Center building was part of wartime Federal Housing, and it was he who sent the keys to me when legal land problems had been resolved. It was Charles Ross, again, who, five years later, volunteered to recommend the construction of Center Park Apartments to the Federal Housing Authority. He was personally involved in every aspect of the project until the building contract was signed. His kindness and patience will be remembered always.

Paul V. Brown was another key person in the first days. As superintendent of Seattle Parks, he convinced his Board to make the old structures available to the Handicapped Club free of charge and without restrictions. His department maintained the grounds; we were responsible for the interior. His interest and support have continued throughout the years, while his wife, *Florence,* equally dedicated, has come weekly with a corps of instructors to teach weaving.

Mayor J. Dorm Braman and the City Council gave support whenever needed; *Mrs. H. Edwards,* as councilwoman, was our firm friend. *Senators Warren G. Magnuson* and *Henry Jackson* gave advice and help at critical points and became honorary chairmen of the Development Fund Drive.

The King County Chapter of the Muscular Dystrophy Association has given regular financial support since early days when meetings were held at the Center. The Seattle Fire Fighters, whose unions nationally espouse the cause of the Association, have given countless hours of volunteer time to remodelling buildings and providing transportation. Zonta Club has been a monthly contributor, also; Beta Sigma Phi Chapters have helped at monthly events and three outstanding youth groups have helped at parties and given transportation for many years: Golden Spurs and Roughriders of Roosevelt High School, and the Spades of Franklin High School. Volunteer drivers, teachers, helpers, are the superstructure upon which all Club programs rest. Enumeration and personal recognition is not possible. However, the most notable characteristic of volunteers is to understand without being told that they are loved, needed and appreciated. They are especially treasured by the Center director!

Substantial grants have made purchase of the present Center building and its remodeling and equipping possible: Boeing Employees United Fund; the Seattle Foundation; *Executive Director Robert Ross* and the Muscular Dystrophy Associations of America, Inc.; the Teachers Foundation; PONCHO; Continental Airlines; Glaser Beverages; the Medina Foundation; *Dr. Richard E. Fuller* and many other firms and individuals. We unitedly and gratefully thank them all. The lives of the physically limited have been immeasurably improved since the founding of the first Handicapped Center.

During the years of developing and directing the Handicapped Center, many people urged me to write about the problems we encountered and how we solved them. But the days and evenings were too filled with the "doing" to allow time for the "recording." Our history, however, lay buried in a pile of clippings, a couple of incompleted scrap books and a file of back issues of the Handicapped Club's magazine, which I have edited for many years. It was this conglomerate that my devoted sister, *Hazel Flagler Begeman*, brought back to her home in Texas, after visiting me in Center Park Apartments for the Handicapped in 1970, and courageously undertook to organize and fuse with her own memories of my childhood. Her daughter, *Jean B. Robitscher,* a journalist, revised and edited our chapters and guided the book through publication in Philadelphia. This triangle of communication stretching from Northwest to South Central to the East Coast has woven together some of the threads of my adventure in a wheelchair. We hope it will be of help to those active handicapped who, today, are awakening to the power inherent in their united efforts.

ADVENTURE IN A WHEELCHAIR

All proceeds from orders will benefit the Seattle Handicapped Center.

ORDER FORM

Please send me..........copies of ADVENTURE IN A WHEELCHAIR at $3.50 per copy postpaid. I am enclosing my check or money order for $..........

Name ....
Street ....
City .... State .... Zip ....

Make checks payable to the Seattle Handicapped Center.
2106 2nd Avenue
Seattle, Washington 98121